THE CALLING

BY
BLAIR GRUBB, MD

THE UNIVERSITY OF TOLEDO PRESS
TOLEDO, OHIO

The University of Toledo Press

Copyright © 2011 by
The University of Toledo Press

The Calling

Library of Congress Control Number: 2011925306
ISBN: 978-0932259-12-7

Brief quotations from these works occur on the following pages:
Joseph Campbell: The Power of Myth
Lance Armstrong: Every Second Counts
David Tame: The Secret Power of Music
David Whyte: The Heart Aroused

Book design by Amanda Russell

Project assistance by Tricia Salata

www.utoledopress.com

DEDICATION

To Barbara Straus, MD: wife, mother, physician, teacher, dancer and soul mate.

TABLE OF CONTENTS

FOREWORD

A physician has the privilege of interacting with other people in a way few others in modern society do. Patients bring to the physician the history of their lives, including their greatest fears and deepest secrets. The physician sees life at both its most difficult and triumphant moments. During the last 30 years I have had the honor and privilege of sharing in my patients' lives. I have watched people face illness, disability and death with a nobility of spirit that leaves me in awe. Listening to them has helped me understand my own life more clearly. In these pieces I recount those stories (as best my memory can recall) that have filled and greatly enriched my life, stories of myself as well as of ordinary men, women and children who find themselves in extraordinary situations. And I hope that you will find within their tales the inspiration and example of how to live in the face of difficult times and experience the courage and resilience that can be found within each of us.

Blair P. Grubb, MD
Toledo, Ohio 2011

ACKNOWLEDGEMENTS

A book is often the culmination of the efforts and influences of many people. I begin by offering my deepest thanks to the many patients I have had the privilege of caring for, who have inspired me both with their stories and their strength in the face of illness. I would also like to thank the late Sy Furman, MD, who encouraged me to write a regular column for the medical journal PACE. In addition I offer my heartfelt thanks to Joel Lipman and the staff at The University of Toledo Press for making this book a reality, and to my children Helen and Alex, whose lives continue to give meaning to my own. But most of all I want to thank my wife, Barbara Straus, MD, for being my muse, an endless source of support and inspiration in my life, without whom I would have accomplished little.

Grateful acknowledgment is made to the editors of the following periodicals and journals where these essays first appeared: Wiley-Blackwell Inc., *PACE*, *Pen World*, The American College of Physicians, and *Annals of Internal Medicine*.

THE CALLING

THE CALLING

*"And he went up, and lay upon the child, and put his mouth upon
his mouth, and his eyes upon his eyes, and his hands upon his hands ...
and the flesh of the child waxed warm."*

—*II Kings 4:34*

FROM THE VERY first I liked him. Paul was a bouncy, broad-smiling, 5-year-old, trusting and innocent. Born with a D-transposition of the great vessels, he had undergone a Senning repair not long after birth. All had been well for years when suddenly he would feel a pounding in his chest and then lose consciousness. The episodes were becoming more frequent and lasting longer. Through Holters and EP study we found he had atrial flutter and sick sinus syndrome. We placed a pacemaker and started him on drug therapy. The episodes stopped.

Young Paul soon became my favorite patient. I looked forward to his visits, where he would jump into my arms, hug me and kiss me on the cheek. He would present me with pictures he had painted, and I would present him with a pen or mug advertising some product. "How's my little buddy?" I would ask as he charged into clinic.

"How's my big buddy?" he would respond as he bounced into my arms. Then, one morning when Paul was 7, I received a stat call to the emergency room. Paul had collapsed at school, a paramedical squad was bringing him in. He was in full arrest; I was there the moment he arrived. The code team, with me directing, worked like a well-oiled machine. Everything went like clockwork, except that Paul wasn't coming back. As the moments wore on I began to feel a growing sense of desperation, which shortly became a sense of panic. I ordered more magnesium to be given. As CPR continued onward and almost an hour had passed, my thoughts began to run wild. "Oh God," I pleaded in my thoughts, "Please not this one. Not him," I began screaming in my mind. "Paul, don't die!"

Suddenly, without even realizing it, tears welling up in my eyes, I was screaming out loud, "Paul, don't die! Oh please don't die!" The code team was shocked at my outburst, and one of my colleagues put his hand on my shoulder saying, "I think I better take over." Yet, no sooner had the words left his lips when someone shouted, "Hey, there's a rhythm!" We looked at the monitor. Slowly at first, then with increasing frequency, QRS complexes started to appear. "There's a pulse!" one of the residents cried out. "I've got a pressure!" said another. Within moments his vital signs had stabilized. Then, for what seemed like an eternity, no one spoke, me staring at Paul, and they staring at me. Suddenly, Paul began to move and gag against the endotracheal tube. He opened his eyes, turned his head and looked straight at me. The head nurse gasped, dropped her clipboard to the floor and made the sign of the cross. The resident who had first felt a pulse, a young Arab, looked pale, and uttered, "Allahu Akbar" (God is Great), while my colleague muttered over and over, "My God, My God ..." I took Paul's hand, leaned over to kiss his forehead, stroked his hair with my hands and wept.

Shortly thereafter he was moved to the ICU, extubated, and made a full recovery. For the next several weeks I was the focus of a number of good-natured jokes, the principal one being that before anyone could end a code they had to page me to come and yell at the patient not to die. After a while, people began to forget the event. After all, they said, it had just been coincidence, the code team had done well, the drugs just needed some time to work. Perhaps, perhaps … but those of us who were there will somehow remember it differently.

I spoke with Paul that next day after the code. He was still groggy, yet hugged me tightly, I asked if he could remember anything that had happened. He sat still for a moment, collecting his thoughts. "It was dark, and I was floating, like I was underwater or something. I wanted to move but I didn't know where."

He paused for a moment. "Then I heard someone calling my name, and then I was moving toward it and it got lighter and lighter." His little boy eyes stared deep into me. "It was you who called me, wasn't it?" "Yes, Paul," I replied, "It was me." "We're still buddies, right?" he asked. "We're still buddies," I said, and held him tight.

That was all many years ago. Most of the people who were there that day have moved on to other positions, other places. But Paul and I are still here, and we're still buddies. He has blossomed into the fullness and energy of young manhood, while the lines on my face have grown deeper, and my hair continues to turn gray. When I saw him last in clinic we spoke of cars, colleges, and careers. He proudly announced to me he would choose a pre-med program. "How did you happen to choose that?" I inquired. "Oh," be replied, "Let's just say it's a calling." And at that, we both laughed.

TO SAVE A LIFE

He who saves a single life
it is as if he had saved
an entire world ...

—*The Talmud*

IT HAD BEEN a bad night. Admissions had occurred one after the other and the beeper went off incessantly. The pediatric intern who struggled to handle a dozen problems at once was exhausted. Changing careers had been difficult for her, going from the artsy world of modern dance in New York to the gritty reality of medicine in an inner city hospital. She never thought that it would be this difficult, but she was determined to keep going. The first rays of dawn appeared. The beeper went off once again, this time calling her to the ER. A 15-year-old young woman had tried an unsuccessful suicide attempt. Psychiatry had already seen her and felt it was just a "gesture," but suggested that she be admitted to Pediatrics for observation. The intern sighed and did a history and physical while the psychiatric resident assured her that suicide precautions were unnecessary. After her admission to the floor was complete, the intern tried to shake off her fatigue and prepare for morning rounds.

Suddenly, she heard the ward nurse scream. Looking up, she saw that the adolescent that she had just admitted had climbed through a window and was walking across the flat tar roof to the edge of the building, six stories above the ground. In a moment, the intern was through the open window. Her dancer's body coiled and sprung across the open roof instantly. She caught the girl just as she was going to jump, but the girl's momentum was such that both were starting to go over the building. The intern struggled to hold on to the girl, bracing her legs against the brick ledge. Within a few moments, multiple nurses and physicians arrived (they had called a code) to pull the two of them back from the edge of oblivion.

Later, after the adolescent was transferred to a psychiatric floor and things had calmed down, 1 rushed over to the intern. "Why did you do that?" I asked. "You could have been killed." She looked at me for a long moment and slowly said, "I had to. If I would have let her go, I could not have lived with myself."

The brilliant social commentator and mythologist Joseph Campbell once became fascinated by episodes such as this, asking, "How is it that a human being can so participate in the peril or pain of another that without thought, spontaneously, a person sacrifices his own life for another? How can it happen that what we normally think of as the first law of nature and self preservation is suddenly dissolved, even for a perfect stranger?"

Campbell found his answer in the writings of the philosopher Schopenhauer, who centuries ago asked the very same question. Schopenhauer's response was that such an event represents a sudden realization that you and the other are one, and that you are but two aspects of life itself, that our separateness is only an effect of the way we experience things under the external constraints of space and time. It is irrational, but that's the point. All compassion, all sympathy is irrational. Love is irrational, yet it defines our humanity. You can see this every day all around you with people doing selfless acts of kindness to and for each other. Once you see this, states Schopenhauer, you will see the truth of your own life.

I looked into the face of the intern, which seemed to glow with a special radiance. I reached out, took my wife into my arms, and held her tight.

THE LAST SUPPER

*T*HEY HAD ONCE been lovers. In the years before our meeting in medical school, my wife during her youth had pursued a career in modern dance in New York City. There, in the artsy world of Greenwich Village, she met Jim, a young dynamic artist and student who struggled to overcome the crippling effects of having been born with spina bifida. Drawn together by their mutual exuberance for life and art, they lived a bohemian existence together. Over time, her increasing fascination with science and medicine and his with finance and business caused them to slowly drift apart. Her departure for medical school, and our subsequent meeting and then marriage, did not end their friendship, and over the ensuing three decades they kept in close touch. In time Jim and I became good friends as well, often trading books and music. Years later, Jim found love again and my wife and I served as the best man and matron of honor at his wedding. Jim pursued a very successful career in investment and decided to fulfill his lifelong dream of retiring early, returning to his native Virginia to once again pursue art. He bought a large tract of wooded land, moved into a small cottage on the property, and began to design the dream house he had always wanted to build. Once it was finished he would have us visit and serve us "a grand supper." He seemed truly happy, but wanted our visit to wait until the new house was complete.

Then, suddenly, he began having difficulty walking and using his left arm. Alarmed, he sought medical attention. The diagnosis left us dumbfounded; multiple tumors were present in his brain. I helped make arrangements for him to be seen at one of the country's top medical centers; the biopsy confirmed our worst fears: an inoperable glioma. Aggressive therapy for a glioma prolongs life by little more than a year at best. He returned home in a profound state of despair. He took a gun from the cabinet, loaded it, and let it sit on his lap.

"Wouldn't it be better to end it now, quickly, and avoid the inevitable slow pain and suffering of a terminal illness?" He held the gun, and sat silent, staring into the woods, waiting, his finger resting on the trigger. Suddenly, a magnificent stag emerged from the forest into the clearing, its antlers held high and proud. Jim took his finger off the trigger and set the gun down. "No," he thought, "I did not spend a lifetime struggling against illness, against spina bifida, to give in now." He would fight and even if he lost he would have at least faced death head-on, with pride, like the stag from the forest.

His condition deteriorated quickly, despite aggressive chemo and radiation therapy. He elected to stay at home, close to his devoted wife and the woods and its animals. He desperately wanted to see my wife one last time and share with us the supper he had long promised. Just before we flew down, his condition worsened and upon our arrival he was confined to a wheelchair, looking wasted, barely conscious and unable to speak. Yet when he heard my wife's voice, he opened his eyes, looked at her, and with a barely perceptible motion gently squeezed her hand. My wife burst out crying and hugged Jim tightly. We spent the day there with Jim and his wife, sitting, talking and sometimes crying. Then, as Jim had wanted for so long, his wife began to prepare us dinner. The four of us sat for what would be Jim's last supper.

The oddness of the scene was difficult to convey. My wife, Jim's wife and I sat around the table, talking and enjoying an excellent meal, while Jim sat at the table frozen in his wheelchair, unable to speak. But we treated Jim like another member of the table; we spoke to and about him, as my wife carefully fed him small amounts of yogurt and water. He was with us. We celebrated his life, his accomplishments and the funny stories that occurred over the course of a lifetime. My wife held Jim's hand and recounted fond memories of three decades past, of Central Park, Sunday papers and building gardens in abandoned lots. Jim would drift away, only to lift his head back up and give a knowing glance to tell us he was present. Finally evening passed into night and we helped Jim's wife get him to bed.

Their cottage was quite small so we had booked a room at a nearby hotel. We both fell into a fitful sleep when a phone call came with the news that Jim had died not long after our parting, as a man at peace with himself. We returned to the cottage to wait with Jim's wife until the funeral home came to remove his body. His body was later cremated and his ashes scattered in the woods he came to love.

So often today we sequester the dying, shutting them away in hospitals or hospices, afraid of them as they serve to remind us of death itself. Yet frequently what the dying most desire is the presence of family and friends, to make peace with the past, and the chance to say goodbye. Having faced a lifetime of disability with courage and fortitude, Jim chose to face death with an equal amount of courage and resolve. I think of Jim now as my wife and I walk through a wooded area near our home. A beautiful stag has emerged from the forest into a clearing, and it holds its antlered head high against the evening sky.

A RIVER OF LIGHT

I DIDN'T KNOW what to say. Mr. Hill just woke up from a week-long coma-like state, brought on by the prolonged resuscitation that he had undergone to revive him from an aborted sudden death episode. He had arrived at the hospital in a deep coma, and I painted a rather bleak picture concerning his chance for recovery to the family that was present. Oddly, they did not seem overly upset at Mr. Hill's current predicament; indeed, they approached his potential demise with a thinly concealed sense of enthusiasm.

Puzzled by the family's behavior, I learned from the nurses in the intensive care unit that Mr. Hill was a well-known business man and investor, known for his ruthless practices, who bought and sold companies with a complete disregard for the people whose lives he manipulated. Married multiple times, his infidelity, alcohol abuse and explosive temper were the stuff of legend. He seemed to have a particular flair for foreclosures and evictions. He was at a local courthouse seizing the assets of a young family (bankrupted by a child's illness) when his cardiac arrest occurred. With each passing day, neurology gave him less and less chance of recovery.

As we were in the process of removing the ventilator, we were shocked to find that Mr. Hill had started breathing on his own. Then, little by little, he made a slow progressive recovery. At first, it appeared that he would suffer severe neurological impairment; he acted like a small child. Then suddenly, he woke up and cried. The nurses paged me and I came to speak with him. Mr. Hill's words virtually flooded out of his mouth: he wanted to tell me about where he had been; he wanted to tell me about "the light." While I had spent a career dealing with sudden death survivors I had never had anyone describe a near death experience to me before.

In great detail he described a sudden feeling of floating, then hovering above his body and watching the paramedic's resuscitation efforts on him. He then described being drawn upward through a passage to a great source of light, "A River of Light" as he called it, where he felt that he was outside the confines of normal time and space, a place that words could not describe. Then, in an instant, he relived the sum of his life, not only from his perspective, but from the perspective of others as well, and he found himself sorely lacking. Then, with great reluctance, he felt himself being drawn back down through the same passage back to his body. I sat silent by his bedside as he spoke, unsure of how to respond.

An estimated 13 million people throughout the world have reported having a near death experience. The term near death experience (NDE) was first used by Raymond Moody in his 1975 book *Life after Life*, and is defined "as a distinct subjective experience that individuals sometimes report after a near death episode, which includes situations in which a person clinically died and was brought back to life, as well as circumstances where death is likely or expected, such as military combat."

While each individual's description of an NDE varies, they tend to be remarkably similar. It begins with an out-of-body experience with the individual observing the attempts at his or her own resuscitation, followed by passage to a place of light associated with a sense of peace and tranquility. Often there is a review of or accounting for the actions of one's life, a process (experienced as either pleasure or agony) followed by the return of the person to his or her body. While debated as to whether these are life after death confirmations or merely elaborate postanoxic hallucinations, there is little debate as to the effect of an NDE on those who report them.

Mr. Hill awoke as a different man who said that he now recognized aspects of the divine in each and every person. The family had little idea how to relate to this radically different person who now smiled, laughed, seemed at peace with himself and said he no longer feared death. His business associates and certain family members demanded that he undergo a psychiatric evaluation. After an hour of conversation, the psychiatrist concluded that he was one of the sanest people he had ever met. He underwent placement of an implantable defibrillator and was later discharged from the hospital.

Mr. Hill's subsequent transformation was akin to something out of Charles Dickens' *A Christmas Carol*. He gave up his previous business practices and set up a large foundation to support charitable causes. He personally sought out the people he had wronged and made amends with each of them. He remarried one of his previous wives and became a faithful husband. He supported every church, synagogue, mosque and temple in the city, saying that each religion was a reflection of the divine. When later he died from end-stage heart failure, he departed as a man at peace with himself. He was hailed as a community benefactor and good citizen.

Since then I had two other patients reporting an NDE, and in each the description was the same and the effect on their lives similar. Irrespective of why NDEs occur, the process seems to represent a cycle of death and rebirth that transforms the ordinary person to a state that some have referred to as the "hero," who now returns to help those around him. I once dismissed these descriptions, but now sometimes I wonder. I have just been asked to see a young woman who suffered a cardiac arrest due to hypertrophic cardiomyopathy, who has just regained consciousness after spending days in a coma, and all she can seem to talk about is having seen a wondrous light.

FINDING PRIVATE REIMER

*T*HERE DID NOT seem to be anything special about him. An elderly man suffering from Alzheimer's, Mr. Reimer had been admitted from a nursing home to the hospital in-patient service with pneumonia and congestive heart failure. Pale and shriveled looking, he would blankly stare out into space. The only thing he ever said was "I'm cold" over and over again. His family had placed him on "Do Not Resuscitate" status and asked us to mainly keep him comfortable. Our service was full of desperately ill people and while attending to his needs, our attentions were frequently focused elsewhere. On rounds, our time with him was usually short, and his constant reply to any question was "I'm cold."

That is except once. As we filed in to the room one morning on rounds, the television was on at full volume, and Mr. Reimer was staring blankly in its direction, seeming to look through it rather than at it. There was a special program on the television concerning the opening of the World War II memorial in Washington. They had been showing colorized films of combat scenes from the Atlantic and

Pacific theaters in tribute to the many brave men and women who served during that horrific conflict.

As we gathered round his bedside to examine him, I suddenly noted his expression change. Within moments it was as if a different man had suddenly appeared, his eyes now sharp, focused on the television screen in front of him. As I turned to look at what had caught his attention, I saw that they were showing grisly photos and film clips of the intense fighting that had taken place in the islands of the Pacific. Almost before realizing it, I turned and asked Mr. Reimer, "Were you there?" He turned his head, looked at me directly in the eye, and to my utter shock began to speak.

"They didn't tell us what we were going into. They didn't tell us how the Japs had fortified the island. The first guys off the boat were cut to pieces by machine gun fire. I made it up the beach and was knocked flat by an explosion. I felt something hit me in the side. It was another guy's leg that had been blown off. A couple of the landing craft had been hit and exploded and a thick black smoke covered the area, making it hard to see me. I crawled forward and saw the Japs were firing from a pocket in an outcropping of rocks. I took one of my grenades and threw it and it bounced off the rock right into the pocket. It must have set off their ammo or something 'cause the whole place exploded in a huge fireball, throwing bodies everywhere. I ran up the hill and one of the Japs popped up in front of me and I shot him in the face. As I turned another lunged forward with a bayonet and I moved fast enough that he just grazed my side. His momentum made him fall on the ground and I shot him in the back of the neck. I turned him over; he looked like he was fourteen."

Mr. Reimer kept speaking, in a voice both clear and mournful, his eyes moist with tears, the words almost pouring out describing the carnage that took place. We had other patients to see, the students were supposed to leave for their conference, beepers went off. Yet no one moved or said a word. Finally, he seemed to exhaust himself, his head lowered, the blank glassy stare returned. After a few moments, he said, "I'm cold." I placed my hand on his shoulder and said, "Rest now," then left with the group to continue rounding.

Afterward, the attitude of the residents toward Mr. Reimer dramatically changed. Two of the interns were from the Philippines and the resident was Chinese (from Nanking to be exact). They had grown up hearing stories of the horrors of the Japanese occupation, and had been ingrained with a deep respect for those who had fought for their liberation. Their treatment of him went from one of indifference to one of near reverence. He went from being referred to as "the patient with Alzheimer's" to "Mr. Reimer." The day nurse (whose father had also fought in the Pacific) paid particular attention to him and even brought in a knit blanket from home to cover him with. Mr. Reimer however had no further "awakenings," slowly slipped into a coma, and died with his family gathered by him.

When I finally met Mr. Reimer's daughter and told her what had happened, she shook her head in disbelief, saying that her father had almost never mentioned the war, and that the only thing she knew was that he had been a private in the Marines. She also said that he suffered from a lifetime of intermittent depression, insomnia and nightmares. She paused, "I wish I would have known" she said, cried, and went to tell the rest of her family.

Psychiatrists who study the effect of combat on veterans have long known that the single most psychologically devastating aspect of war is not the fear of being killed, or the loss of one's comrades, but rather the knowledge that one has taken the life of another. There is something deep within us that rebels against the killing of a fellow human being, no matter how just the cause may be. Close combat leaves deep emotional scars that never really heal. It is said that Alzheimer's is a disease of memory, the growing plaques infiltrating and disrupting the neurons that permit recall of the past. But perhaps, it may sometimes strip away the conscious suppression of memories that are just too painful, too disturbing, too agonizing to recall. Yet those memories are there, lurking just below the surface waiting for the right moment to suddenly reappear.

While Alzheimer's had stolen the man his family had known and loved, in the end it helped them regain something that had long been lost, it helped them find the frightened, courageous, and troubled young man who had once been Private Reimer.

A GLASS OF
AMONTILLADO

I RARELY MAKE HOUSE calls, in fact, almost never. But then Madame Bonterin was not your usual patient either. It was a cool summer's day that had passed to that magic time just before dusk that the French refer to as "Le Crepuscule." I walked quietly through the flower garden that seemed to burst forth with color and fragrance from every corner. There I found her, an old but sturdy woman, elegantly dressed, sitting in a reclining lawn chair under a tree. "Bonjour," I said as I approached. Looking up from her book, she eyed me with an impish smile. "Bonjour," she replied. She certainly did not look to be 93 years old. "Ah, my friend, please sit." I pulled up a chair next to her and began my examination. Peripheral edema, basilar rales, and an S3 gallop all pointed to an exacerbation of her congestive heart failure.

Normally, I would hospitalize someone in this condition, but I knew that with Madame Bonterin I would be wasting my breath. We had done this many times before. I sighed, and reached into my doctor's bag (which I specifically stocked for this visit). I placed a small intravenous line in her forearm and carefully injected a dose of diuretic.

In a very short time she said she felt better and disappeared into the bathroom. When she reappeared, she was holding what appeared to be a bottle of wine and two glasses. I was about to protest that it was not a good idea to drink in her state, but thought better of it. After all, she had made it this far without heeding any of my advice. She showed me the bottle which had the name "Amontillado" written on it. "Cognac is for lovers, Amontillado is for friends."

Her face was radiant. Despite her years she seemed to display an ageless beauty, a quality that French women have always seemed to master. I was fascinated by her and the air of mystery that always seemed to surround her. She had lived through two world wars, fought with the French resistance, escaped from a Nazi prison and had outlived three husbands. Art and literature filled the stately country home where she now resided. I stood saying that I really should be going, but she stared directly into my eyes and said, "You will rush yourself into an early grave." I paused a moment and sat down again.

She poured two glasses and sat next to me. "You Americans, always in such a hurry," she said, shaking her head and taking a long slow sip of wine. "If you hurry pleasure then you will miss all the subtle sensations that make the experience worthwhile," she continued. "In the end you will scarcely recall what it is you've done. Speed, you see, is a way of forgetting." We sat for over an hour, speaking of the past, the world, families and wine. She had a fondness for Amontillado. "At first it is undrinkable, only when exposed to heat and the elements does it become something unique and wonderful," she said as she finished her glass. "So too with people. It is the stresses of life that give us our unique characteristics."

The wine worked its magic upon me and I felt myself relax, sensing, as if for the first time, the beauty of the moment, the garden, the setting sun and the songs of the birds. Finally I rose, bid her goodbye and left. Many months later I learned that she died quietly in her sleep, her death being the same as she had lived her life, on her own terms. Not long afterward, I was contacted by a local law firm. Madame Bonterin had included me in her will; she left me a case of Amontillado.

I think of her now as I sit on the back porch of my house, surrounded by family and friends. There is no particular reason for our gathering, other than to be together on a cool summer evening. As the children play, the adults sit, talk, tell stories and laugh, while each of us sips slowly on a glass of Amontillado.

THE COLOR OF SILENCE

$\mathscr{H}$ E LOOKED SO alone. A Japanese executive from a major firm, Mr. Tanakya was in town for a business meeting when he was seized with severe chest pain. Taken to our hospital's emergency room where I was the cardiologist on duty, I was concerned about the diffuse ST segment changes present on his ECG. He had already been seen by one of the cardiology fellows who advised him that a cardiac catheterization would be needed, but he refused. Several months prior to this, I had been to Japan as a visiting professor, and in the process became fascinated by Japanese culture and traditions.

Upon entering his room, I bowed politely and presented him with one of the business cards in Japanese. He bowed from his bed, took my card and studied it for a moment, then made a gesture for me to sit. Slowly and respectfully I explained what I thought was wrong and why he needed a catheterization. A man accustomed to making decisions, he pondered the matter for a few moments and then gave his consent. The catheterization demonstrated a blockage in his left main coronary artery, a condition that would require open heart surgery to correct. However, he was noted on x-ray to have a possible pneumonia, and as his chest pain had now subsided, he was admitted to the coronary care unit for antibiotic therapy until his infection had passed.

As luck would have it, when he called his family in Japan, he learned that his wife had been admitted to a hospital there with severe abdominal pain. His daughter was in the last weeks of a difficult pregnancy and had been advised not to travel. He would have to face this alone. He sat in his bed immersed in an air of melancholy.

I felt sorry for him and tried to think of something that would cheer him up. Then it occurred to me. Years ago, my wife had introduced me to the game of Go (called Igo in Japan). Although appearing deceptively simple, it is one of the most complex and intricate games ever devised. Two players take turns placing small black or white stones on a flat wooden board marked with 19 horizontal and 19 vertical lines that form a grid. Originating in China almost 2,500 years ago, it makes chess seem relatively new by comparison, and is far more demanding (despite a $1.4-million prize, no supercomputer has yet been able to beat even a mildly competent amateur Go player). I had played some and owned a Go set, and thought I might cheer Mr. Tanakya up by playing a game or two with him.

The next day after rounds, I showed up with the game and asked Mr. Tanakya if he would like to play. He gave me an amused look.

"You know Go?" he asked.

"Yes," I replied naively and set the board up, hoping to play a relaxing game with him. I got annihilated so quickly that it made my head swim. I asked him to play a second game, and got beaten more promptly than in the first. He smiled and told me that Go was one of his passions (he was a player at the second dan, a considerable level) as well as that he was a devotee to the Zen arts and thought. I felt like an idiot, thanked him for the game and left. Yet that night, I realized that having a Go master here was a unique experience. So the next day I went to his room, bowed and politely asked if he would teach me how to play Go. He wrinkled his forehead.

"Why?" he inquired.

"Because I realized that I know nothing," I said.

He thought for a long moment, looked up, and gestured for me to sit. Thus began a strange relationship that continued throughout his long stay in the hospital. By day I was the physician and he the patient, by night he was the teacher and I the pupil. Each evening after work, I would show up in his room, bow, sit and play. Go is a game so simple that the rules take half an hour to learn and yet so complex that it takes a lifetime to master. It ranks with calligraphy, painting and music as one of the four essential Zen arts of Japan. When we would start a game, his melancholy would evaporate and be replaced by a certain sense of austerity. It has been said that "if chess is a battle then Go is a war." The board begins bare, like a clean slate. The goal of each player is to outline and take territory by placing his stones on one of the board's 361 intersections (compared to 64 for chess). As opposed to our first match, in each game I was given a handicap, commensurate with his level of skill and my inexperience. He would counsel me prior to each move, "Don't attack the densest place" and "Be patient," and "Silently observing often is best." His memory was astounding; he seemed to remember every move I had made in every prior game and would comment on them.

"Remember the mistake you made in game four," he would say. I could remember hardly anything about game four, and much less which of my multiple mistakes he was referring to. Nonetheless, I slowly became better (meaning, it took longer for him to beat me). I became obsessed with Go, trying to map out moves in my mind by day and dreamt of Go by night. However, slowly Mr. Tanakya showed me that Go (and by extension, life itself) is less about winning than it is about the game's own inherent beauty. He tried to convey the game's intrinsic sense of harmony (or "Wa") that arises out of apparent discord, and with it a sense of humility and respect for nature. I came in on my off days and on weekends to play. We even played the day after his bypass surgery, despite his obvious pain and discomfort (which was the only time I actually came close to beating him). A Go master cannot describe how to play the game in purely logical terms, and therefore he had me contemplate several Zen style "koans" (word challenges) to help me think differently (for example, "What is the sound of one-hand clapping?"). In the West, we would call this "thinking outside the box." Tradition is that a teacher will choose a unique koan for each student. I waited for mine. Each time I would ask, the reply was the same.

"Focus on the game."

Finally, our time together came to an end, and he was well enough to make the trip back to Japan. I gave him a fountain pen with his name engraved on it, for which he expressed his deep appreciation. I took him to the front door in a wheelchair, where a limousine was waiting to take him to the airport. As he rose to get into the car, we both bowed, and he thanked me for my care in the hospital and with an impish look added, "Your learning has begun well." I was expecting to be given my own koan, but with that he entered the car and was gone.

Several weeks later, I had to go to the post office to sign for a package that had come from Japan. It contained a beautiful Go set as well as a set of Japanese calligraphy brushes and paper, along with a note consisting of a single line: " Consider, the color of silence."

I smiled and laughed to myself. To be honest, I'm still thinking.

THE ACCIDENT

*I*T WAS, AFTER all, a mistake. It had been one of the worst nights of my residency. There had been so many admissions that I had virtually lost count, and I was barely able to keep up with the needs of my own patients, much less all the other ones I was cross-covering. I was desperately rushing to finish checking labs and ordering tests before hurrying off to morning report. Later that day I was struggling to fight back fatigue and finish attending rounds when I received a page to report to Radiology immediately.

"Oh great," I thought, "Now what's wrong?" However, upon my arrival, I was the sudden focus of congratulations and pats on the back.

"Great pickup!" they said. "Look at that," one of the radiologists said, pointing to films from an upper GI series hanging on the viewbox.

"A small bowel tumor, classic appearance!" I stood there dumbfounded; I had no idea what they were talking about. I picked up the chart and leafed though it. Yes, I had ordered the upper GI, but it wasn't my patient. Then I realized what had happened. In my haste to keep up with everything the prior evening I had ordered an upper GI on the wrong patient!

Looking closer at the chart, I learned that the patient was a priest and director of a local Catholic college. He had been complaining of cough and fever, as well as nonspecific malaise and therefore was admitted to the hospital for an evaluation. The upper GI showed a leiomyosarcoma of the bowel that luckily had not spread and he was operated on the next day. The surgeon paged me to the operating room to show me saying, "You really saved this guy's butt. I've never caught one of these this early before." I was too embarrassed to say anything, so I nodded my head politely and walked out. I didn't tell a soul what had happened.

The hectic pace of residency quickly resumed and the incident was soon forgotten. About a week later, I was paged to the surgical floor. When I returned the call one of the nurses informed me that one of the patients wanted to speak with me. I told her that I didn't have any patients there. She replied, "It's a priest, and he's quite insistent on speaking with you." I froze and felt a deep sinking feeling in the pit of my stomach. In a near trance-like state I slowly made my way to his room. As I entered I had a sudden urge to throw myself at his feet while saying, "Forgive me, Father, for I have sinned," but instead I quietly introduced myself and took a seat by his bed. He was a distinguished looking man in his late fifties with piercing eyes that seemed to stare directly into my soul.

"Were you the one who ordered the test on me?" I nodded my head and said nothing.

"Why?" he asked.

"It was . . . an accident," I stammered. I told him everything, the words almost pouring out of me, a relief to finally tell someone.

He appeared pale and said nothing for a long time, the two of us sitting in utter silence. After a while he finally spoke.

"The last several months have been something of a spiritual crisis for me. I had begun to question how I had spent my life, and the very core of my beliefs. I was offered a new and important position, but I didn't feel capable or worthy of it. Then, I began to feel ill and I was going to turn the offer down." He paused. "Since the surgery my symptoms seem to have disappeared. I now know what I should do. You see, my son, I believe there are no accidents. When they came to take me for the test I knew that something was amiss, yet at the very same time I felt deeply that I had to go."

He seemed to sit more erect in bed and his voice gathered force. "The day before I had prayed for some sort of sign to guide me, and now I understand that you were chosen to be its instrument." As he spoke I felt the hairs on the back of my neck rise and a strange sensation came over me.

The noted theologian Rudolph Otto used the term "numinous" to describe such events. To him, numinosity described the feeling that somehow we are undeniably, irresistibly and unforgettably in the presence of the Divine. It is our experience, even for a moment, of something that transcends our human limitations.

I sat there stunned, not knowing what to say or think. The priest smiled. "Such talk troubles you, doesn't it?" he said. I told him of my own inner struggles trying to reconcile reason and faith in the context of my own religious tradition.

"Ah," he replied. "One of your people grappled with such questions long ago. I will introduce you to him."

My beeper summoned me. As I rose to leave, he asked that I wait for a moment and sit on his bed. He placed his hand upon my head and said, "I offer you my thanks in the words your people once taught us: 'May the Lord bless you and keep you, may his face shine upon you and be gracious unto you, may he lift up his countenance upon you and give you peace.'"

Several months later I was called to the hospital's mailroom to sign for a package that had just arrived for me from Europe. I was shocked to see that it had come from the Vatican. Opening it I found that it was from the same priest, except instead of father his title was now monsignor (a "knight" of the church) and a special assistant to the pope! Inside was a short note that said, "As you once helped me through my spiritual turmoil, may this aid you through yours." Enclosed was a beautiful bound English translation of the great physician and philosopher Moses Maimonides' monumental work on the struggle between faith and reason, *The Guide to the Perplexed*, complete with commentaries. I walked to the small patient garden next to the hospital entrance, sat, and heard the soft songs of the birds and caught the smell of the spring blossoms in the clean air.

I sat holding the book and was lost in thought for a long time. It was, after all, just a mistake. Wasn't it?

I CHOOSE TO GO
GENTLE

"Do not go gentle into that good night, rage,
rage against the dying of the light."
—*Dylan Thomas*

I WAS A NEW attending physician, fresh out of a cardiology fellowship, my first month running the intensive care unit. One of the first patients admitted to me was Jennie, a clear-eyed, attractive woman in her late forties, suffering from severe heart failure, which in turn had caused her kidneys and liver to begin to fail. Hopelessly ill, she had been transferred to our university hospital to see if she would qualify for a heart transplant. Almost immediately after she arrived she suffered a cardiac arrest and through a superhuman effort we managed to get her back. She required constant attention; I practically lived by her bedside. Twice more she arrested and twice more we snatched her from the jaws of death. A former nurse and school teacher, she was a widow with two grown children. During quiet times she read poetry, the work of Dylan Thomas among her favorites.

After extensive testing, the transplant team informed me that she was not a suitable candidate. Too many other organs were involved and she probably would not survive the stress of the surgery. I broke the news to her and her family as gently as possible. "I figured as much," she said. "I know all of you have worked so hard." She reached next to her bed and brought out a small package. "I want you to have this," she said. "The nurses told me that you like pens."

Opening the package I found a blue lacquer Targa fountain pen. I expressed my heartfelt thanks to them. She then looked straight at me and said, "I ask not to be resuscitated if I arrest again. It has been enough fighting. It is my time, and I choose to go gentle into that dark night." Her sons nodded their agreement. "Of course," I said, trying to fight back the tears that somehow seemed to come to my eyes. With the very same pen I wrote "Do Not Resuscitate" on her chart. Not more than an hour later she was dead.

To this day I use the pen, its presence a reminder of those bonds that link each of us together. That life is both beautiful and mysterious in ways that are sometimes beyond comprehension, and that even in death there can be nobility. There are times when it is better to go gentle into that dark night and quietly bid farewell to the fading light.

— AWAKENING —

*T*HERE WERE SO many admissions that night that I had begun to lose count—and my temper. A seasoned intern, I had learned well the art of the quick, efficient workup. Shortcutting had become a way of life. Morning was coming and with it, my day off. All I wanted was to be done. My beeper sounded. I answered it. I heard the tired voice of my resident say, "Another hit, some 90-year-old gomer with cancer." Swearing under my breath, I headed to the room. An elderly man sat quietly in his bed. Acting put upon, I abruptly launched into my programmed litany of questions, not really expecting much in the way of answers. To my surprise, his voice was clear and full and his answers were articulate and concise. In the midst of my memorized review of systems, 1 asked if he had ever lived or worked outside the country.

"Yes." he replied. "I lived in Europe for seven years after the war." Surprised by his answer, I inquired if he had been a soldier there.

"No," he said. "I was a lawyer. I was one of the prosecuting attorneys at the Nuremberg trials." My pen hit the floor. I blinked.

"The Nuremberg trials?" He nodded, stating that he later remained in Europe to help rebuild the German legal system.

"Right," I thought to myself, "some old man's delusion." My beeper went off twice. I finished the examination quickly, hurried off to morning sign-out, and handed over the beeper.

Officially free, I started out the door but suddenly paused, remembering the old man, his voice. His eyes. I walked over to the phone and called my brother, a law student, who was taking a course on legal history. I asked him if the man's name appeared in any of his books. After a few minutes, his voice returned.

"Actually, it says here that he was one of the prosecution's leading attorneys at the Nuremberg trials." I don't remember making my way back to his room, but I know I felt humbled, small and insignificant. I knocked. When he bid me enter, I sat in the very seat I had occupied a short time before and quietly said, "Sir, if you would not mind, I am off duty now and would very much like to hear about Nuremberg and what you did there. And I apologize for having been so curt with you previously." He smiled, staring at me.

"No, I don't mind." Slowly, with great effort at times, be told me of the immense wreckage of Europe, the untold human suffering of the war. He spoke of the camps, those immense factories of death, the sight of the piles of bodies that made him retch. The trials, the bargaining, the punishments. He said that the war criminals themselves had been a sorry-looking bunch. Aside from the rude awakening of having lost the war, they could not quite understand the significance of the court's quiet and determined justice or of the prosecution's hard work and thorough attention to detail. The Nazis had never done things that way. So moved had he been by the suffering he encountered there that he had stayed on to help build a system of laws that would prevent such atrocities from happening again. Like a child I sat, silent, drinking in every word. This was history before me. Four hours passed. I thanked him and shook his hand, and went home to sleep.

The next morning began early, and as usual I was busy. It was late before I could return to see the old man. When I did, his room was empty. He had died during the night.

I walked outside into the evening air and caught the smell of the spring flowers. I thought of the man and felt despair mixed with joy. Suddenly my life seemed richer and more meaningful, my patients more complex and mysterious than before. I realized that the beauty and horror of this world were mixed in a way that is sometimes beyond understanding. The man's effect on me did not end there. Despite the grueling call schedule, the overwhelming workload, and the emotional stress of internship, something had changed within me. I began to notice colors, shapes and smells that added magic to everyday life. I learned that the gray-haired patients that I had once called "gomers" were people with stories to tell and things to teach. After nearly two decades, I still look to that night, remember that man, and reflect on the change and privilege we have to share in the lives of others, if only we take the time to listen.

SUNDAY IN THE PARK WITH GEORGE

If I am not for myself,
Who will be for me?
Yet if I am only for myself
What am I?
And if not now, when?

Hillel, Pirke Avot 1:14
—*The Talmud*

*G*EORGE WAS DYING, and all of us knew it. A generous, kind, and caring man, his recurrent admissions for heart failure made him a frequent sight on the wards, and everyone's favorite patient. A retired sports broadcaster, he would enthrall myself and other residents with stories of Brooks Robinson and Johnny Unitas. Baseball had always been his favorite sport and he had played in the minor leagues before going into sportscasting. He had grown up in the neighborhood and everyone seemed to know him and would call him by name. Multiple heart attacks had left him with severe congestive heart failure, and with each admission he seemed to grow ever more weak and frail. Finally, his heart failed so badly that he would gasp for breath despite a facemask of oxygen and multiple intravenous medications.

Yet he hung on; the will to live was strong within him. He would often gaze out the window from which you could see a corner of a park where he often played as a boy. I was a resident then and found that his deteriorating condition filled me with a growing sense of frustration and hopelessness. I wanted desperately to be able to do something to ease his suffering. When I asked if there was anything that I could do for him, he looked straight at me and said, "Yes, there is. I want to go to the park."

I stood dumbfounded. Go to the park? In his state? Ridiculous! Yet he persisted and I came to realize that it was a dying man's last request. When I asked the attending physician if somehow we could take him to the park, he looked at me with an expression of disgust and said definitely not. Yet somehow I could not get the notion out of my mind and I began to secretly plot with the nurses (who adored George) about how we were going to take him to the park. I knew I was potentially risking my career, but somehow it didn't seem to matter.

We planned to do it on the coming Sunday when I had off and when a different attending was cross-covering. When the day came, two nurses who were supposed to go home stayed and together with one of his daughters, we carefully eased George into a wheelchair and gathered together oxygen bottles, IV infusion pump, intravenous bags, tubing, and medications. Then with a sense of growing apprehension (and at the same time, adventure) we made our way to a freight elevator where we hoped to draw little attention. As we wheeled George out a side door into the street, people stopped and stared in disbelief at the sight of two nurses, a doctor and another woman pushing a patient in a wheelchair hooked to multiple machines. We paid no attention to anyone and pressed forward toward the park. For his part George was in high spirits and would at times exclaim, "Yee-ha!" as we bounced along the bumpy sidewalk.

It was a beautiful summer day and the park was green, lush and full of children. We stopped a little way into the entrance, near a pagoda-like building with a pond around it. George was lost in thought for a time then told us that he had proposed to his first wife at that very spot. We then wheeled him over to the ball diamond where a group of children were enthusiastically engaged in a baseball game. George was delighted, and joyfully recounted tales of when he had played as a boy in the same field. His eyes twinkled with delight as the cool breeze brought with it the smell of hot dogs and barbecued chicken. As I looked at him I suddenly realized that I wanted to be a boy again, but this time together with George as a boy. I wanted to run with him through the fields, ride together on our bikes and try to hit his famous fastball. I wanted to taste the wondrous energy of youth again with him as my friend. I sensed the decades that separated us in age were artificial barriers with little meaning.

After a while we had to leave. George reached down and pulled dandelions from the grass and held them up under his oxygen mask to inhale their fragrance. His face seemed radiant and content. He thanked us over and over again.

When we returned the attending physician and head nurse were furious and my worst fears were realized as all of us were suspended. When George and his daughter heard what had happened to us, his son-in-law (a prominent attorney with a major law firm) called the attending and the head of the hospital to inform them that he and his firm would be representing us legally if they continued with our suspension, and that he would bring to bear "the full weight of all resources available" to him in our defense. The suspension was lifted the next day, and no one spoke of it again.

Thereafter, George appeared to be a man at peace with himself despite his deteriorating condition. He died a week later with his family and many of the housestaff and nurses at his bedside. I wept like a child for a man who, in another time and another place, I would have wanted as a friend. After the funeral, none of us could quite think of what to do. Suddenly one of the nurses had an idea. We all drove to the same park where we had taken George only a short time before, went to the same ball diamond, and still in suits, ties and dresses, began to play baseball.

DRIVING ELIJAH

> *"He has told you, O man*
> *what is good, and what the Lord*
> *requires of you: only to do justice,*
> *to love goodness, and to walk humbly*
> *with your God."*
> —*Micah 6:8*

IT HAD BEEN a bad week. While trying to recover from surgery, I received news that because of an unexpected huge increase in the cost of labor and supplies, the grant that I had worked so hard to get would run out before my research project could be completed. Simultaneously, several faculty members announced that they would be leaving, making a difficult work schedule even worse. I was in a bitter mood when I drove to the community center to pick up my son after his basketball practice. As we scurried out the door to get to his piano lesson, a small white haired old man, hunched over a walker, approached us and said, "Could you please give me a ride home?" He had apparently missed the last seniors' bus of the day and was stranded. Before I could utter a word my son (who was eight at the time) virtually shouted, "Sure we can!" I sighed. We were on a tight schedule and this was the last thing I needed. But he looked so frail and pitiful that I reluctantly agreed.

As I pulled the car around, my son carefully helped him off the curb, and then together we eased him and his walker into the back seat. I was somewhat surprised when he mentioned where he wanted to go, as it was a fairly nice part of town. When the man asked what my son's name was, my son (in his usual exuberant manner) proceeded to tell him not only his name but also his school, where we lived, his favorite sports, and that my wife and I were physicians!

Before the man had a chance to say a word, my son quickly added, "Daddy's upset cause his grant money's gone." "Really?" the man replied, after which he asked what kind of research I did. In the course of my attempts at explanation he asked several, surprisingly insightful questions. I asked if he had been involved in research in the past. "No," he replied somewhat wistfully, stroking his beard, "I worked for a bank." I was about to ask another question when he suddenly announced, "Ah, we're here." I pulled over and my son and I helped him out of the car. He no longer seemed quite as old or as frail as he once did. Indeed, his white beard seemed to glisten and his blue eyes seemed to twinkle. He expressed his thanks and shook my hand firmly saying, "Don't give up, things always seem to turn out all right." I did not feel comforted. As we whisked off to my son's piano lesson he looked at me and in his youthful innocence asked, "Could that have been Elijah?"

I laughed. In his Sunday school class he had listened to the many folktales about the biblical prophet Elijah. Legend has it that he perpetually wanders the earth, each time in a different guise or form (usually of someone helpless or in need), to test the goodness of men and women and reward those he deems worthy. "Those are just stories," I said, and fell silent, putting the incident out of my mind.

Several weeks later when I arrived at work the office of the college's Foundation called to say that they had received an anonymous grant of $10,000 to be used for my research. I was shocked and asked if he knew who had given it. He replied that the lawyer from the bank handling the donation had said he was under strict orders not to reveal its source. I put down the phone with a feeling of elation when I suddenly remembered the old man. A strange sensation came over me and I sat in silence. "No," I said to myself, "it couldn't be." Nonetheless, I called the community center to see if anyone knew who the old man was. No one could remember anyone like that. I left work and drove to the center and looked and asked around about the man, but to no avail.

With the anonymous grant we were able to complete the project. To this day I have no idea if the old man and my sudden deliverance from failure were in any way connected. The rational part of me keeps saying they aren't, but somehow I can't help wondering.

When I told my son what had happened he jumped up and down and smiled from ear to ear. "See, Dad," he exclaimed, "we were driving Elijah!"

DAYBREAK AT ANGKOR WAT

J DIDN'T LIKE HIM at first. Although John was only in his late fifties, he was a physical wreck. Overweight and suffering from years of alcohol and cigarette abuse, he wore dirty clothes and shoulder-length white hair that reeked of stale beer, cigarettes and old sweat. His pale skin was covered with cuts and bruises, and his legs were grossly swollen with edema. He had a long history of emphysema and end-stage congestive heart failure, the latter of which was worsening due to his uncontrolled chronic atrial fibrillation. Given his worsening condition (and his history of poor compliance) we elected to implant a permanent pacemaker in him followed by an atrioventricular nodal ablation (as was popular in those days).

He complained about everything: the physicians, the nurses, the food, the bed. He would suddenly explode in anger and spew forth a stream of curses directed at any and everyone. It was a busy day and he was the last person that I wanted to put up with. He continued to complain as we prepared him for his pacemaker, saying that the procedure room was too cold. Finally we were ready to begin. I had the nurses give John some intravenous narcotic for sedation, hoping that he would finally be quiet. While he didn't stop talking, he did stop complaining and his voice took a softer, more positive tone. He started talking about the Vietnam War, of being in an elite Special Forces unit that had been sent to secretly fight in Cambodia. He criticized the government's handling of the war and the way veterans of that conflict were treated afterward. At last he seemed to fall asleep and for a moment I savored the thought of finishing the pacemaker in peace.

Suddenly he awoke and roared, "Do you know anything about the Angkor Wat temple?" "Not really," I said from behind the surgical drape that separated us, trying to focus on placing the pacemaker lead in an adequate place. John thereafter launched into a lecture. While on patrol in the jungle he had come upon one of the greatest monuments ever built by mankind, indeed the largest religious structure in the world. Built in the first half of the 12th century when the Khmer civilization was at its peak, Angkor Wat is an enormous temple symbolizing a mythic mountain, with five interconnected rectangular walls and moats representing heavenly mountain chains and the cosmic ocean.

He was overwhelmed by its huge ornate towers and miles of carved stone sculptural reliefs. He stumbled upon it at daybreak and said that it seemed to suddenly rise up out of the ground, like a supernatural creation of the gods. He stood dumbfounded, unable to move, overwhelmed by the sheer size and beauty of it. He spoke of its grand halls and intricate carvings, and said that while he stood there the war seemed both distant and petty. He spoke unendingly about the temple complex for the remainder of the procedure.

The following day, when he was brought back for his ablation and once again sedatives were given, he launched into a series of stories about Angkor Wat, Southeast Asia and the war. Everyone present listened intently to his recollections of friends and lives lost, of having been a prisoner of war and his subsequent torture and escape. In the process my image of him slowly changed from a street drunk to a person whose life had been ravaged by war, and I realized that his broken body still held a decent man inside.

The procedures proved effective, his condition stabilized, and he was later discharged. His discussions of Angkor Wat had piqued my interest and I ordered a book of photographs of the site. The pictures showed a monumental site of awesome beauty, and I wondered how much more grandiose it must be to see in person.

When John returned to the pacemaker clinic he looked somber and again smelled of cigarettes and alcohol. When I gave him the book as a gift his face was suddenly transformed, his hard features softened and his eyes became moist. He held it close to his chest, closed his eyes and uttered a barely audible "Thank you." I later received a letter from him saying how much the book meant to him, how he was trying to turn his life around, and how he was looking forward to seeing me again. Several months later I learned that he had died in his sleep. At his funeral I was told that he had received a Bronze Star for bravery in combat, had been married four times, and had passed away holding the book I had given him close to his side.

I keep the letter from John in a special place in my desk, as a reminder that things are often deeper and more profound than they first appear. That patients labeled as "difficult" were nonetheless people with stories to tell and lessons to teach, who experience joy and suffering just as we do.

Since that time I've read further about and seen more pictures of Angkor Wat, and John was right, it is one of the true wonders of the world. And maybe someday, somehow, I'll be able to stand there and see what he once did, the day breaking at Angkor Wat.

—— "MY DEAR CHILD" ——

I'VE ALWAYS DREADED these days. Once a year, to evaluate the progress of residents and interns, one of the faculty observes them performing a complete history and physical on a new clinic patient. These tend to be tedious, drawn out and often boring affairs as the residents try to impress the observer by asking the patient every conceivable question. To make matters worse, I somehow had to squeeze this into an already busy clinic schedule.

The perky young woman who was the intern I was to evaluate and I entered the exam room to find two Asian women, one older and one younger. It turned out they were Cambodian. The older woman was the patient; the younger woman, her niece, had come to translate. She had been having palpitations, the niece said. Having to go through a translator was making this take even longer than usual. The patient, however, seemed an intelligent woman with an air of refinement about her. She had been educated in France and had taught school after returning to Cambodia. The intern asked if she was married. Her niece replied that she was a widow. After a number of other questions the intern asked how many times she had been pregnant. There was a pause. Four times, was the translated reply. "How many are now living?" was the next question the intern asked. The niece hesitated, looked at me, and then slowly translated the question. Upon hearing it, the older woman hung her head, as tears began to roll down her cheeks, and uttered a barely audible reply. "None" the niece said. The intern sat in shocked silence. "How?" she stammered.

The answer was gut-wrenching. Between 1975 and 1979 the Khmer Rouge took over Cambodia and initiated one of the worst nightmares of modern history. Hoping to "cleanse" the country of outside influences, they brutally tortured and murdered over two-and-one-half million people (almost 20 percent of the country's population). They singled out the educated professionals for "special" treatment. She had hidden, together with her infant son, in the attic of their home as her husband—a pharmacist—and three other children were dragged into the street and machine-gunned as she watched helplessly. Later she slowly made her way through the jungle over several weeks, scavenging for food and hiding from the Khmer Rouge. Her infant son later died of fever and diarrhea shortly after she got to a refugee camp in Thailand.

Her story was interrupted by a knock on the door. The nurse was informing me that the patient in the next room was becoming upset at having to wait so long. I excused myself and went next door to explain.

I had known the old woman in the next room for a long time. Mrs. Mayer sat with her walker, with a sour look on her face. I started to tell her why we were late, why the woman next door needed more time, why I couldn't just leave, why ... then I stopped short. The number tattooed on her left arm reminded me. She had been at Auschwitz. Her first husband and child had died there. We stared at each other for a long moment. "Go back to her," she said firmly. As I left the room, I realized Mrs. Mayer was following me. I started to protest but she would hear nothing of it. "She doesn't speak English," I said, "only French and Cambodian." Mrs. Mayer ignored me, went in, sat next to the woman and started speaking to her in French. I could not tell what they were saying. After a few minutes both women were crying, sharing a kind of grief that only they could know. Mrs. Mayer then wrapped her arms around the woman and uttered over and over, "Mein teier kind, mein teier kind (my dear child)..." The woman's niece, the intern and I stood by silently, unable to do or say anything. After a time they calmed down, exchanged phone numbers, and Mrs. Mayer said she would call her later.

The nurse again popped in to say the rest of the patients were getting upset at having to wait so long. Mrs. Mayer stood up and said, "Doctor, you finish with this woman, I will speak to the people in the waiting room." I protested, but she went anyway. I'm not sure what she said to them, but no one said a word about being late afterward.

After clinic was finished I met with the intern to review her evaluation. While she had managed to keep her composure during the history and physical, after discussing the case she broke down and started to cry. "How can people do such a thing?" she managed to say between sobs.

How indeed? How could the world watch as six million Jews and nearly five million others were slaughtered by the Nazis? How could the world watch as Stalin presided over the deaths of nearly 20 million people and Mao's cultural revolution killed an estimated 60 million? Where was I when this woman's family was murdered? Studying for finals? Worrying about grades? I shook my head, unable to answer her question.

When I arrived home that evening my young daughter and son ran to greet me. The sight of them made the two women's grief even more palpable. I held them close to me and softly uttered, "My dear children."

THE SACRIFICE
OF ISAAC

*I*T HAD BEEN a bad night. I was on my first clinical rotation as a medical student and the OB/GYN service was swamped with patients. I had patiently assisted the residents with over a dozen deliveries, and the chief resident had promised that the next delivery would be mine. My excitement and anticipation quickly evaporated when the person who would be my first delivery appeared: a 300-pound woman, nine months pregnant, who arrived on the back of a Harley Davidson motorcycle. The man who was driving the motorcycle was of equal girth with a beard to his waist and whose head was covered with a red bandana. It was also apparent that she had not bathed in, well, a long time. By the time we got her in the door she was already contracting and a pelvic exam revealed that she was fully dilated (it also revealed a tattoo on her left buttock that said "Satan's slave"). "Stay with her till we get a delivery room ready," the resident yelled as he disappeared down the hall, "and don't let her push!" I tried to explain to her that she needed to calm down, to focus on breathing. But she wasn't listening, she was crying. "If it is a boy I want him called Isaac," she sobbed. "That was my daddy's name." I tried again to calm her, saying she could name the child whatever she wished. She wasn't listening. "I want him to have a better life than me, to have a chance at being somebody," she said through her tears. She stopped suddenly and said, "Oh my God, it's coming!" "No, wait!" I yelled, "Don't push!" She pulled her legs up and gave one tremendous grunt and I abruptly found myself performing my first delivery. Actually it was more like a catch, the baby literally popped out into my reluctant arms; I was struggling to keep from dropping the child when I noticed it was a boy. At that moment the resident returned and started yelling that I should have waited until he had returned. I tried to explain what had happened, but was interrupted by the mother's sobs and her demands to hold the child. We carefully cut the cord and placed the child in its mother's arm. "Oh Isaac," she cried, "you're going to be somebody, you're going to be better than me." Her words seemed to baffle me, but my attention was diverted to delivering the placenta. The resident felt that the child looked pale and called the neonatologist to see him. The pediatrician wanted to admit the child to the nursery for observation. The mother reluctantly parted with the infant, crying over and over, "His name is Isaac." She seemed inconsolable. I finally got a chance to start an IV on her, gave her some fluids and a sedative and moved her to the recovery area. I wanted a chance to speak with her, find out why she was so upset at a time when most women are filled with joy. But no sooner had we moved her to recovery than our attentions were drawn to another patient who arrived in active labor who was bleeding profusely. When I finally returned to the recovery area to check on the woman I was shocked to find the bed empty and the IV dangling in the air: she was gone. The staff looked everywhere for her to no avail; she had disappeared without a trace. It was then that I realized that we knew nothing about her except her name, Sara Smith. The police were notified, and baby Isaac stayed in the nursery for days while they searched in vain for his mother. The child was made a ward of the state and soon adopted. I later heard that when the adoptive parents heard the story of the child's birth they decided to honor the mother's request; they named the child Isaac.

Now in retrospect, the woman's behavior was understandable. In her mind she was making the greatest sacrifice possible for the good of the child she knew she could not raise. Now, three decades later, these memories flood back into my consciousness. Today a married couple I know who have been trying to adopt a child for years are bringing home the infant that they had yearned for over so many years. It is a beautiful little boy, and they have named the child Isaac.

WASHING THE DEAD

*T*HE RING OF the telephone jolted me from sleep. After a somewhat hectic night on call I had tried to retire early. In a half-dazed state, I answered the phone. I recognized the voice on the other end instantly. He said, "It is time. Meet us there in half an hour." I put down the phone, dressed quickly, and began to reflect on what I was about to do.

He had been a good man, generous, kind and well liked. He had been my patient for a long time, one of the first patients in whom I had placed an implantable defibrillator. Slowly, over those years, he changed from patient to good friend. We had faced many crises together over the years, and somehow his failing heart always managed to pull through. When he was diagnosed with lung cancer, both of us knew he would not last long. On the last clinic visit prior to his death, he looked at me and said, "You have been a good friend over these years. I have only a little time left. Would you be part of the Chevra Kadisha after I die?"

I froze, speechless. The Chevra Kadisha, or Holy Society, is a voluntary group in the Jewish community whose sole purpose is to prepare the body of the deceased prior to burial. It is the greatest of honors to be asked to do such a thing, and almost before realizing it I said, "Of course."

Over the following months the other members of the group prepared me. Tradition dictates that the funeral take place as soon as possible after death; thus, there is often little notice. We meet in the parking lot of the funeral home. We greet each other and converse quietly until the other members of the group arrive. Together as we enter the funeral home the mood is restrained, as each of us has a set responsibility to attend to.

The dead must be treated with the greatest of respect at all times and our duties performed quietly and meticulously. We gather together, wash hands and recite a blessing. Then, with the greatest of care, we wash the dead. Ever so gently, avoiding any sudden or jarring movements, his body is sponged clean. Odd, to see the man I had known in life in the stillness of death. Even though my mind often drifts back to memories of him in life, I try to focus on washing the same torso where the implantable defibrillator I once placed still lies. When the cleansing is complete, his body is carefully given a mikvah, a ritual bath, for symbolic purification. Then after he has been fully dried, we dress him only in a plain white linen shroud.

As we do this, I recall a passage from the Talmud that says, "When a child is born his fists are clenched as if to say, 'All this will be mine.' Yet when a man dies his hands are open, as if to say, 'I bequeath this all to you for I can take nothing.'" Finally his body is placed into a plain wooden casket and a prayer shawl is wrapped around him. During this entire time my heart has been pounding and beads of sweat have covered my forehead. Somehow this has been more stressful than performing a procedure on a living patient.

Now finished, we gather and ask for forgiveness from the soul of the departed (for each of us realizes that our minds have not been totally focused during the process of preparation). On occasion, one of the group will stay behind, sitting at the side of the casket reciting verses from Psalms until the burial is complete, making sure the body of the departed is not disturbed. On the drive home I cannot help but wonder why I was so nervous beforehand, and why I now feel such a feeling of satisfaction (as well as relief). I sense that I have fulfilled a sacred obligation, a debt that the deceased can never repay.

Perhaps my anxiety was because of the distinct contrast between this ritual and the attitudes I have witnessed toward the dead during my medical career. While in my residency the attending physicians would often utter phrases like "death with dignity," their actions all too frequently fell short of that ideal. We have tended to see death as some kind of failure on our part as physicians, rather than the natural or inevitable process it is. We retreat from the dead, and the families of the dead, as soon as possible, unsure of what to say or do. Death seems to be one of the few subjects that remains forbidden in American society, and physicians, for the most part, seem little prepared to deal with it.

Several weeks later another patient (of a different ethnic and religious tradition) whom I had known for years died after a prolonged illness. This time, instead of leaving the family after they were informed, I stayed as they mourned and then escorted them to the patient's bedside. After a moment of silence I turned to leave, but one of the family members said, "Please, don't go yet, doctor." She took my hand in hers, as the rest of the family gathered around the bed. Then, in the clearest and most beautiful voice she began to sing "Amazing Grace."

I noticed the usual noise of the ward had stopped, as everyone present, physicians, nurses and visitors, patiently stopped everything for a moment, just to listen.

IT SHOULD ONCE AGAIN SEE LIGHT

$\mathcal{S}$EVERAL YEARS AGO, a physician from southern France contacted me. His granddaughter had taken ill with a disease that baffled the physicians there. He called after reading several of my articles on disorders of the autonomic nervous system. His granddaughter's symptoms seemed to match those I had described, and he asked me if I could help. I readily agreed, and for many months, I collaborated with the child's French physicians by telephone and by fax, directing their diagnostic testing. At last we came to a diagnosis, and I prescribed a course of therapy. During the next several weeks, the child made a seemingly miraculous recovery. Her grandparents expressed their heartfelt thanks and told me to let them know should I ever come to France.

In the summer of 1996, I was invited to speak at a large international scientific meeting that was held in Nice, France. I sent word to the physician I had helped years before. Upon my arrival at the hotel, I received a message to contact him. I called him, and we arranged a night to meet for dinner.

On the appointed day we met and then drove north to his home in the beautiful southern French countryside. It was humbling to learn his home was older than the United States. During the drive he told me that his wife had metastatic breast cancer and was not well, but she insisted upon meeting me. When introduced to her, I saw that despite her severe illness, she was still a beautiful woman with a noble bearing.

I was thereafter treated to one of the most wonderful meals I have ever eaten, complemented by the most exquisite of wines. After dinner, we sat in a 17th-century salon, sipping cognac and chatting. Our conversation must have seemed odd to the young man and woman who served us because it came out in a free-flowing mixture of English, French and Spanish. After a time the woman asked, "My husband tells me you are Jewish, no?" "Yes," I said, "I am a Jew." They asked me to tell them about Judaism, especially the holidays. I did my best to explain and was astounded by how little they knew of Judaism. She seemed to be particularly interested in Hanukkah. Once I had finished answering her questions, she suddenly looked me in the eye and said, "I have something I want to give to you." She disappeared and returned several moments later with a package wrapped in cloth. She sat, her tired eyes looking into mine, and she began to speak slowly.

"When I was a little girl of 8 years, during the Second World War, the authorities came to our village to round up all the Jews. My best friend at that time was a girl of my age named Jeanette. One morning when I came to play, I saw her family being forced at gunpoint into a truck. I ran home and told my mother what had happened and asked where Jeanette was going. 'Don't worry,' she said, 'Jeanette will be back soon.' I ran back to Jeanette's house only to find that she was gone and that the other villagers were looting her home of valuables, except for the Judaic items, which were thrown into the street. As I approached, I saw an item from her house lying in the dirt. I picked it up and recognized it as an object that Jeanette and her family would light around Christmas time. In my little girl's mind I said, 'I will take this home and keep it for Jeanette, till she comes back,' but she and her family never returned."

She paused and took a slow sip of brandy. "Since that time I have kept it. I hid it from my parents and didn't tell a soul of its existence. Indeed, over the last 50 years the only person who knew of it was my husband. When I found out what really happened to the Jews, and how many of the people I knew had collaborated with the Nazis, I could not bear to look at it. Yet I kept it, hidden, waiting for something, although I wasn't sure what. Now I know what I was waiting for. It was you, a Jew, who helped cure our granddaughter, and it is to you I entrust this."

Her trembling hands set the package on my lap. I slowly unwrapped the cloth from around it. Inside was a menorah, but one unlike any I had seen before. Made of solid brass, it had eight cups for holding oil and wicks and a ninth cup centered above the others. It had a ring attached to the top, and the woman mentioned that she remembered that Jeanette's family would hang it in the hallway of their home. It looked quite old to me; later, several people told me that it is probably at least 100 years old. As I held it and thought about what it represented, I began to cry. All I could manage to say was a garbled "Merci." As I left, her last words to me were "Il faudra voir la lumiere encore une fois"—it should once again see light.

I later learned that she died less than one month after our meeting. This Hanukkah, the menorah will once again see light, and as I and my family light it, we will say a special prayer in honor of those whose memories it represents. We will not let its lights go out again.

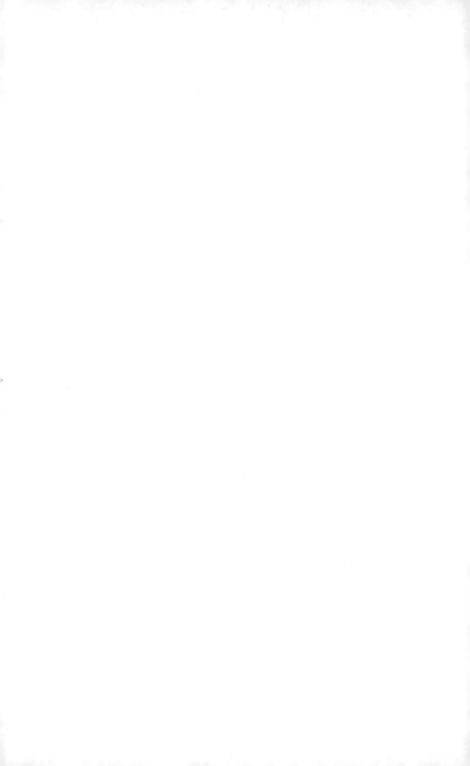

—— GENERATIONS ——

"What profit hath a man of all his labor that he takes under the sun?
One generation passes away, and another generation comes. But the earth
abides forever ... All rivers run to the sea, yet the sea is never full ..."
—*Ecclesiastes 1:3-7*

*M*Y FATHER WAS, among other things, a maker of signs. My youth was spent surrounded by the smells of paint, the feel of different brushes, and the markings of ruler and square. Now, as I reach to pick up a brush, I stop and for a moment, my mind drifts back to childhood, to the day my father first taught me to paint.

"Before you begin," he would say, "frame the piece in your mind, picture its details. Then, mark the lines carefully, they will guide your hands."

"Hold the brush like this, turning the tip slightly upward," he would instruct as he held my hand with the brush in it, guiding its motion.

"Bring the stroke down firmly but carefully, make each part flow." Each letter had its own character, its own personality. Each had to be perfect, yet joined into the whole. The spacing had to be varied to give the word balance. No matter what the sign said, or where it went, it was a reflection of the painter. Slowly, I learned the art he had perfected, for among his peers he was considered a master.

My father was a lover of music. The sounds of Benny Goodman, Glenn Miller and the other masters of swing would course through our house or car and my father's pleasure at hearing them was almost palpable. So, even now, when the sound of the big bands or swing comes across the radio, without warning, a feeling of sadness arises within me.

My father was a lover of leather. He admired that it kept out the cold winds, that it was tough yet smooth, and that it got better with age (he would often wink at my mother and say "Remember son, only wine, leather and women get better with age.") Now, as I wear the jacket that was once his favorite, the soft touch and gentle smell of it floods my mind with memories and a wave of emotion passes over me. Somehow at these odd moments, I deeply feel his presence around and within me.

A father remains a father, even when the weight of years renders him frail and old, and even when he lives only in your memories. Perhaps his death has made his existence even more meaningful to everyone whose life he once touched. I think of that now as I gather the brushes and paints, and the ruler; these objects now becoming a cherished reminder of my regard for him, even though my father is now gone.

Today is a special day. My daughter has asked me to help her with the lettering of her school project. She has asked me to teach her to paint a sign.

"Draw the lines straight," I say as my eyes somehow begin to moisten. "They will be your guides."

"Hold the brush like this," I intone, my voice crackling slightly with emotion as I take her hand to guide her strokes. I show her how to make the top of the 's' smaller than the bottom, how to space the 'i' closer to keep the perspective right, curve the top of the 'o' slightly more than the bottom, and flare the leg of the 'r' outward to give it balance.

"Yes," I tell her as her hand moves gently across the surface, carefully making each letter, "bring the stroke down firmly."

I smile as I watch her, and feel a tear slowly making its way down my cheek.

"That is good, let the paint flow." All this I show her, for among other things, I am her father, and I too am a maker of signs.

--- REQUIEM ---

*J*ANUARY 30, 1944, Anzio Beach, Italy. The Allied invasion of central Italy is bogged down in a deadly game of mutual slaughter. The numbers of dead on both sides are immense. The Allies are desperate to break the stalemate. The generals think they can break through the German lines near the town of Cisterna, but they need more information on enemy positions and strength. A crack commando unit under the command of an aggressive young sergeant is chosen to go in. Their mission is secret. Only the top command knows of it, and radio silence will be maintained.

The sergeant leading the men is worried. Having lied about his age and enlisted at 17, he has fought his way across North Africa and the invasion of Sicily. The men under him are like his family, and he doesn't like the idea of taking them this far behind enemy lines. He worries that his own cousin will be with him, a man he loves like a brother.

Before dawn they move slowly and silently through the war-ravaged hills. The sergeant is where he always is, out in front. He has ordered his cousin to be in the rear of the advancing group, figuring he will be a little safer there. The sergeant's eyes survey the surreal scene of burned out buildings and blackened trees; his ears strain to hear through the eerie silence.

An Allied spotter with a telescope on a far hill faintly sees them moving. He is unsure whether they are Allied or German, and he radios back to his commander in a forward artillery group. The lieutenant who receives the message is young and brash. Fresh out of training and son of a congressman, he has been in combat for less than a week. Usual procedure would be to radio Central Command and check to see if any Allied units were operating in that area. He does not check. He wants to prove himself. He orders the whole artillery battery to fire on the area.

The sergeant is moving his men forward slowly and carefully, trying to keep track of each one. Suddenly, the world explodes. Seemingly, everywhere at once, shells are hitting and blowing the tiny valley they are in apart. The Allies and Germans use different artillery shelling patterns. He instantly realized the shells are coming from his side. He turns and screams at the radioman to make contact and tell them to stop, but as the words leave his lips, the man disappears in a billow of flame and a cry of agony. He orders his men down, to try and take cover. He runs back to check on the wounded. Suddenly, he feels he is flying through the air, then, darkness.

When he awakens, there is stillness all around him. Smoke covers the area and the smell of death is everywhere. He tries to stand, but cannot. His left leg is shattered and blood soaked. His left arm dangles useless at his side. He screams, but hears nothing. He drags himself along and then stops. In front of him are pieces of his cousin's body. He hangs his head and cries. He stops, there is a voice calling. Yes, a voice, calling for help. He drags himself over to the sound. He finds one of his men there.

"I'm cold," the man whispers. A man drained of blood gets very cold. There is not much that a man with a shattered thigh can do, but a man whose chest has been torn to ribbons by shell splinters can do even less. The sergeant wraps his arm around his comrade, and slowly and painfully begins to drag him back toward the allied lines. The pain is nearly overwhelming, but he does not stop; his only focus is to pull the wounded man along. There is no time, only pain and motion.

The lieutenant now radios Central Command and learns he has just shelled a company of U.S. troops. A squad is sent out. They find the wounded sergeant dragging one of his men nearly a mile from the side where the shells hit. All the others are dead. The sergeant sees the men coming. "You bastards!" he screams, then again darkness.

When he awakens, the first thing he notes is the smell of the antiseptic. He tries to move but cannot. His right hand and both legs are encased in a plaster cast. His head is bandaged. Only his right arm is free. Seeing his movement, a nurse calls out, and several doctors come. He has lain in this hospital, comatose for nearly a month. He hears what happened, and that the man he pulled out has lived. The lieutenant who ordered the barrage was relieved of his command, but was reinstated after several phone calls from Washington. They tell the sergeant he is a hero, that he has been awarded the Bronze Star. But he feels no joy, only anger seething deep within him.

The next day a general arrives. The sergeant will be given a medal for heroism, as if that will somehow heal the wound that festers in his soul. With great pomp and ceremony they pin the medal on his bandaged chest. The sergeant picks it up, looks at it for a moment, and then throws it at the general, striking him in the face. There is shocked silence, and then rapid motion as the general and his staff turn to leave. The rest of the men in the hospital begin to cheer.

The general is furious, and demands a court-martial. But parts of the story have been leaked to the press, so the incident is attributed to "battle fatigue" and forgotten. The sergeant does not forget, and the pain of learning to walk again only deepens the memory. He returns home a hero, but finds no glory in it. He moves away, hoping to somehow start over.

My father seldom spoke of the war. I knew he had been in North Africa, Sicily and Italy, but little else. His answers to my questions were always oblique. He always carried a mild air of melancholy about him that intensified when the war was mentioned. After a while, I stopped asking. He would sometimes awaken at night screaming, and jolt me terrified from sleep. In time I learned to ignore it.

In the spring of 1998, my parents had come for a visit. While my wife and mother took the children to the park, my father asked that I stay behind with him. He wanted to talk to me. I do not know why he chose that moment to break a half-century of silence, but he did. As he spoke, he cried. I had never seen my father cry before. He talked for over three hours, often having to stop and compose himself. When it came time for them to leave, we hugged each other tightly. It was to be the last time I would see him.

On my own, I contacted the military. Yes, was the reply, the events were true. Was the medal awarded taken back? No, it was never rescinded. After several months, I obtained a Bronze Star. I wanted him to have it, from me and from the men of his company.

The medal arrived days before my wife and I were to leave for Europe. At first I had planned to wait until they visited to present it to him. However, a strange sense of urgency seemed to come over me and I decided to mail it to him. With it was a letter, saying how much I loved and respected him, and that this medal was not from the military, rather it was from the American people, the men who served under him, and me. "If you listen closely to the heavens," I wrote, "you will hear the applause of your comrades, for they have long awaited this day."

When we returned home I called. For the second time, I could hear my father cry. Over and over he thanked me. We would talk more when they came out again next month. His final words to me before hanging up were "This is the finest present I have ever received." He told my mother that he felt a sense of peace that he had not known in a long time. A week later, he died.

I stood at the graveside of the man who had been my father. How little I really knew of him and much of what he was will always remain a mystery. I stood for a moment, wiped the tears from my face, and raised my hand in one final salute. Rest in peace father, rest in peace.

ANTHONY'S ASHES

*E*VERY GUY IN the residency program envied him, not to mention most of the senior male physician staff. Anthony (Tony) DeAngelo was the image of a Greek god personified. He was six feet tall, had blond tousled hair, and blue eyes with the muscular conditioned body of an Olympic athlete. His romantic exploits with the nursing staff were the stuff of legend. He was also one of the brightest interns in the program, with an innate ability to sense what was wrong with a patient. He seemed always to be happy. As I got to know him and his past better, his pleasant demeanor surprised me even more. He appeared to have no family. Born to American parents working in Argentina, Tony returned to the United States to live with an aunt after both his parents died in a tragic automobile accident. However, several years later his aunt also died (of cancer), an event that propelled him into a series of foster care programs and facilities. His sharp mind and quick wit won him full scholarships to college and medical school, and ultimately to the same residency as me. He seemed possessed of inexhaustible energy and humor. He had a disdain for pretentiousness, formality and ceremony. "Don't take yourself too seriously," he often said. His long hair, scruffily unshaven face and casual dress drove the senior attending physicians crazy. When one of the attendings ordered him to wear a shirt and tie on rounds, he showed up with a carefully knotted bow tie on top of a tee shirt. He was also a practical joker who could entertain patients by juggling a series of tennis balls, while taking a history. Patients loved him; the difficulties of his own life gave him a deep empathy for the sufferings of others. He loved the open water of the nearby bay. He owned a small sailboat that he spent every free moment sailing regardless of the weather or temperature. On more than one occasion he would say to those of us fortunate enough to go out in his boat with him, "When I die I want my ashes scattered in the bay." We laughed at that; after all, he seemed immortal, possessed of an almost divine stature.

As our internships drew to a close, Tony announced that he had decided to change from Internal Medicine to Surgery. After an unruly party held dockside by his boat, we all said our goodbyes, confident that Tony would charm the surgeons the way that he had charmed us.

Two weeks later, we heard the awful news. Tony had literally dropped dead at a welcome party for the surgical residents and could not be resuscitated. An autopsy revealed that he had suffered from an undiagnosed cardiomyopathy. Those of us who knew him were stunned and overcome with a sense of grief beyond words. Another problem then quickly arose. Tony appeared to have no family, so who would make the funeral arrangements? Our program director quickly took responsibility for the matter, and personally paid for Tony's cremation. It was decided that we would follow Tony's prior wish: his ashes would be scattered into the bay. In order to accommodate all the people who wanted to be present, a large ferryboat (usually used for tourists) was rented for the occasion. When the appointed day arrived, those of us who worked with him (as well as a surprising number of distraught nurses) showed up in suits and formal dresses. Once the boat was out in the bay, we gathered in the open rear area of the boat. Our program director and the hospital chaplain then delivered the kind of formal eulogies that would have aggravated Tony to no end, had he been alive to hear them. There was just something about all this that did not seem quite right.

In retrospect, the whole affair had not been well thought out beforehand. When the time came to scatter his ashes into the water, we all gathered solemnly in the back of the boat. The jar holding his ashes was opened and tilted to let them ride the wind off the back of the boat and into the water. But the winds of the bay are unpredictable and can shift direction instantly. As the chaplain held the jar aloft, the winds suddenly changed, and Anthony DeAngelo's ashes flew back in all of our faces and covered our fancy clothes.

There was a stunned silence that seemed to go on eternally. Then one of the nurses started laughing hysterically. "Hey Tony" she shouted, "just couldn't resist that last joke, could you?" Suddenly the mood changed, the tension of the moment faded and the boat roared with laughter mixed with tears. People embraced, or shook hands. Out of nowhere bottles of tequila (Tony's favorite drink) suddenly appeared. We shed our soiled jackets and ties and dusted as much as we could of Tony's ashes in the water. As the bay churned around us, we let the cool wind blow in our faces and watched the setting sun. Then, until late into the night, we told stories about Tony, and drank toast after toast to him, just the way he would have wanted.

THE FLOWER

"Be a lamp unto yourself. Be your own confidence.
Hold to the truth within yourself.
There is nothing else you need to achieve. Just open your eyes."
—*The Buddha*

THE SUN BEAT down mercilessly on the cinderblock clinic in the small Dominican town of El Valle. Fresh out of medical school I, along with another new graduate from Puerto Rico, worked under a young Dominican doctor who had just finished his residency. We were the only medical care available in the entire region.

Each day, 70 or more people would wait patiently in long lines to be seen. Many had walked miles to seek medical attention and some of the sicker ones had been transported by horse or burro. The numbers of people sometimes seemed endless, and when we finally closed the clinic each evening, the lines were already forming with the next day's patients, who would often wait through the night. We frequently would work 12-14 hours, and yet the lines waiting would seldom diminish. The police would sometimes come around closing time to try and keep order.

One of my first mornings there, a young woman, around 18 years old, entered the exam room with a small infant cradled in her arms. The child was wrapped in blankets (despite the intense heat) with a kerchief around its head. One of the Haitians who would come to harvest the sugar cane crops, she spoke Spanish only haltingly. She placed her child on the exam table and slowly removed the multiple blankets while telling us that the child had had days of diarrhea. Looking at his limp form, I could tell the child was dead. I listened to his chest, but heard no heartbeat.

I called out for Fernando, the Dominican doctor, who came over and confirmed the fact that the child was dead (probably for some time). I tried to explain as best as I could, but the mother refused to listen, repeating over and over, "No, baby still warm." The nurse attempted to gently take the baby from her, but she clutched him even more tightly. Suddenly, she lashed out violently, knocking the glasses off my face. She screamed out something in French-Creole and stormed out of the clinic, still holding the child tightly.

I stood there numb, in a state of shock. The nurse told me that she said she was going to seek the help of a local witch-doctor. Juan, my co-worker in the clinic, saw what had happened and walked over to our nurse. Juan, a large and imposing-looking man, had spent two years in Vietnam and after winning a Purple Heart and Bronze Star for valor, renounced violence and converted to Buddhism. Juan and the witch-doctor had become friends in the short time we had been there, figuring it would be better to work with him than work against him.

Juan quickly scribbled a note and told the nurse to go to the witch-doctor via a back path. As she disappeared I asked Juan, "What did you write?" He uttered a deep sigh and said, "There is a story that the Buddha, after his enlightenment, had a woman bring him her dead child asking if he could restore his life. He replied that she would have to first bring him a cup of mustard seed from a household that had never known suffering. She went from house to house, but could find none that had not known sorrow. She eventually gave up, and buried the child."

He shrugged his massive shoulders. "The witch-doctor is a reasonable man. He will not try to bring back the dead. I asked him to have her bring him a cup of sugar from a family who had not known sorrow." The witch-doctor followed Juan's advice. The woman searched frantically, but there was no such family in El Valle. She eventually gave up, and let the police take the child to be buried.

Later, after the clinic had finally closed for the day, we wandered into the field behind the building. There, we sat on the grass amidst dozens of blooming wildflowers, listening to the calls of the birds, saying nothing. I kept thinking about the child, the mother and the fragility of life here. I felt overwhelmed by a sense of grief and futility, hung my head, and wept.

After some time, I turned to Juan and asked, "So what did the Buddha have to say about life?" In reply he said nothing, reached over and picked a single flower, holding it in front of me. I stared at it and suddenly saw that it was beautiful. At that moment the whole world seemed full of wonder.

— TO TAME A HEART —

I HAD NO IDEA what to do. For months I had struggled in vain to control Stephanie's multiple implantable defibrillator shocks. Once a perky 16-year-old, she suffered a cardiac arrest while sledding, and survived only because of her older brother's determined efforts to give her CPR. After spending several days in a coma she finally awoke, and subsequent studies showed that she suffered from a severe form of Long QT syndrome. When well enough she underwent an implantable cardioverter defibrillator (ICD) placement, was placed on a beta-blocker and sent home. Confident in our treatment, I assured Stephanie and her family that "things would be fine" from this point on and that she might get "occasional" ICD shocks.

I had no idea how wrong I was. Within days she was back in the hospital after experiencing multiple defibrillator shocks, sometimes as many as ten in a single day. At first I thought the device was malfunctioning, but analysis of the ICD showed that every shock had been appropriate, each one terminating an episode of potentially lethal ventricular fibrillation.

I increased her medications but the shocks continued. The hospital telemetry monitor confirmed the appropriateness of each of the shocks; she seemed to be having "storms" of ventricular fibrillation. I tried reprogramming the device, changing her medications; nothing worked. At times her episodes of fibrillation would lessen enough to get home, only to have her return after a flurry of ICD shocks. I called colleagues across the country for advice, added new medications, made more changes in the ICD settings, yet the shocks continued. I racked my brain trying to figure out why her heart suddenly seemed so irritable, why she so often was so perilously close to death.

The experts I called had little to offer. It seemed that every other week she was in the hospital or the device clinic. The frequent shocks took a heavy emotional toll on Stephanie. She sunk into a deep depression and withdrew from the world into herself. She dropped out of school, read fantasy novels, and in a fit of melancholy shaved all the hair from her head. I watched helplessly as the child's life force seemed to slowly slip away.

Then suddenly I heard nothing from Stephanie or her parents. Weeks went by and I had not received a single call about her. Worried, I called her home, but there was no answer. I assumed that she had gone to another center for yet another opinion.

Finally, months later, Stephanie and her mother showed up in my clinic. However, instead of her usual glum demeanor she looked happy and flashed a huge smile as I walked in. She proudly reported that she had not had a single ICD shock in nearly three months. Indeed, analysis showed that she had not had a single significant arrhythmia through the entire period.

How had this happened? Was she taking some new medication? Had she been seen by a different electrophysiologist, who had been able to control what I was not? No, she said, she had not been seen elsewhere. I shook my head. "So what happened to bring this about?" I asked, intrigued beyond measure.

Stephanie blushed for a moment; she said that the minister of her church had suggested that she get some type of pet. Her mother took her to the pet shop and in the process of picking out a puppy she started speaking to a young man her age who was working there. He apparently caught sight of the scar near her left shoulder and said, "Hey, do you have a pacemaker?" "No," she replied cautiously, "it's a defibrillator, why?" "Well," he said, "it looks just like my pacemaker," at which point he pulled open his shirt to show his own pacemaker scar as well as a large scar that ran down the middle of his chest. She learned that he had had surgery to repair a congenital heart problem and was dependent on his pacemaker to live. They immediately took a liking to each other, and had seen each other daily since then. "Did you get the puppy?" I asked. "Oh yes," she beamed, "a beautiful terrier." Somehow, the combination of a puppy and a boyfriend had brought the storms of lethal arrhythmias under control. I stared at Stephanie; she looked the best that I had ever seen her.

I felt bewildered, confused. I almost didn't believe her at first. How could a boyfriend and a puppy have brought under control an arrhythmia that our best efforts had failed to help? I continued to follow Stephanie over the years. She has experienced occasional ICD shocks, but nothing to the magnitude that she once did. She has grown into a lovely young woman, both confident and caring.

I often think about Stephanie. She taught me a powerful lesson: that there are things in life that we cannot measure, that our emotions interact with our biochemistry and physiology in ways beyond our understanding, and that the course of an illness is sometimes as unique as each individual. In few other conditions is the interplay between emotion and physiology as great as in the congenital Long

QT syndrome, where fear and fright may quickly culminate in death.

The cyclist and cancer survivor Lance Armstrong has stated, "You can save someone's life, but what about the quality of that life?" Stephanie broadened my narrow concepts of health and disease. Now I often ask patients, "What do you need most at this moment?" Often it is just a friend or a sympathetic ear; sometimes it is understanding or forgiveness. A wise old adage of medicine advises that it is not sufficient to merely understand the disease; one must also understand the patients who suffer from the disease, their lives, hopes, dreams and fears. Stephanie taught me this by taming a heart that I could not.

That was all years ago. Recently I received an invitation in the mail; Stephanie and the young man she met in the pet shop are getting married.

— THE JUST —

"All things change when we do..."
—*Kukei, The Zen Poems*
8th Century C.E. Japan

H E WAS A good man. I was fresh from fellowship, with a pregnant wife and a small child, and Tom, who lived across the street, was the first one to show up the day we moved to the neighborhood. He was gray-haired with a broad grin, and we had been there only 10 minutes when he introduced himself with a "Hi-yah-there" and a firm handshake. Within moments he was helping us unpack, giving my wife directions to the supermarket, and instructing me on the finer points of lawn care. A retired businessman, he had a down-home humor and good nature that made him like a modern-day Will Rogers.

I soon learned that we were not the only recipients of his kindness. The children in all the surrounding neighborhoods all referred to him as "Grandpa." They would gather round his feet to listen to his stories of the war and life in the Pacific. When anything broke, Tom was the first person you would ask about it. He somehow seemed to know everybody; with a single phone call he could have a repair person there in minutes. When a baseball shattered the glass of the front door, Tom helped my wife pick up the broken pieces, disappeared with the frame, and reappeared later with a new window made of high-impact plastic. When I offered to pay, he only winked; "the store owner owes me a few favors," he said. When there was a local blood shortage, he was the first in line. When a windstorm left the area covered with broken tree branches, he was there to help clear away the debris. When I got too busy to mow the lawn, he did it. He was a regular at the corner coffee shop where he often "held court." If you needed someone to talk to, about anything, he would listen. I marveled at the man. He seemed to be the very embodiment of goodness. But it had not always been so.

One afternoon, sitting on the back porch sipping iced tea, he shared with me that for a long time he had been anything but saintly. Severely wounded in the Pacific campaign of the Second World War, he had lost sight in one eye and hearing in one ear. Often in pain from his wounds, he became a heavy smoker, hard drinker, and ruthless businessman. He was not, as he put it, "a nice man." Yet things changed dramatically one day when he attended the funeral of a friend from his childhood. His friend had been a kind and caring person, beloved by family and friends. Hundreds of people had shown up to pay their respects with heartfelt feelings of grief.

"I realized that if it was my funeral at that moment few people would bother to show up." He paused and took a sip of tea.

"Then the strangest thing happened. Suddenly I realized what I had become: a drunk, cruel brute. It was as if I just woke up from a long sleep."

He stopped smoking and drinking that day, sold his business and devoted himself to the community with a passion that made those who had known him question his sanity.

"I had a lot of lost time to make up for," he reflected. Miserly before, he gave away great sums to charity after what he referred to as "the change." He joined every civic organization in town. His one wish was that at least a few people would someday show up at his funeral.

Yet as good as he was, the years of cigarettes and alcohol caught up with him and he suffered a massive heart attack helping an elderly neighbor clear away a fallen tree. He died the following day. The community was stunned, and my children cried incessantly. On the weekend of the funeral, the bell of a small nearby church next to the cemetery began to ring in a slow rhythmic tolling. On and on it tolled. Slowly, one by one, people stopped what they were doing and began to walk to the graveyard. Stores closed, restaurants emptied, and the playgrounds fell silent. Soon a crowd of over 100 people had gathered around the side of Tom's grave and more continued to come. The police showed up to keep order, but they were not needed. Instead, they joined the throng. As the pallbearers went by, people reached out to touch the casket. People I have rarely seen show any emotion wept openly. The bell continued to toll unendingly till nightfall, and the crowd did not dissipate for hours. I smiled through my own tears as I realized that Tom had gotten his wish.

There is a legend from the Cabala that the world is sustained through the actions of 36 just and righteous people. Referred to as the "Lamed-vovnik" (the 36 or simply "The Just") their goodness sustains our world, and without them all would soon fall into chaos. No one knows exactly who they are, but they are out there, amongst us, sustaining us all. It is said that when one of them dies, their soul passes to another, who then takes the job of "Tikkun," restoring and redeeming the world.

I think of that now as I sit on the porch where I once would spend evenings chatting with Tom, and I wonder to whom his spirit may have passed, for surely he was one of The Just. Perhaps it is someone you know who lives nearby or right across the street, and maybe, just maybe, it is you.

A BLESSING ON THE MOON

I DIDN'T THINK MUCH of it. After all, it had only been a type of innocent amusement. My wife and I had attended an anniversary party for friends at which one of the major entertainments prior to dinner was a group of fortune tellers who read palms, analyzed handwriting, determined horoscopes, or read Tarot cards to predict the future. The Tarot card reader was the most popular. An older, yet still attractive woman, the Tarot reader exuded a sense of serenity and confidence. After turning the cards she would deliver her reading in lighthearted verse, usually predicting that fortune and fame were just around the corner. However, when my turn came and she flipped the cards, a somber look came across her face. She stared first at the cards, and then at me. "Exercise caution at the coming new moon," she said slowly, "for it will bring a blessing, or your doom." She then abruptly stood up and excused herself. I puzzled over her words for a while, and then forgot about them, my mind drawn back into the whirlwind of day-to-day life.

As the days and months went by I became increasingly aware of an uncomfortable feeling deep within my chest. For years I had suffered from esophageal spasm, so intermittent chest discomfort was nothing new to me. Yet there was something naggingly different in character about them this time. It is difficult to describe the feeling, as it was neither a pain nor a sense of pressure.

Even today, I am at a loss for words in attempting to categorize it. How does one describe the color blue or the taste of salt? Words describe shared experiences, and there was nothing in my experience that compared to this. Concerned, I consulted my internist, who promptly ordered a nuclear stress test. I ran on the treadmill far beyond my projected workload, and the electrocardiogram and nuclear images were read as normal. While the rational part of me was reassured, I continued to experience a deep sense of unease.

As the weeks went by the discomfort continued, waxing and waning in intensity, sometimes occurring with exertion, sometimes not. Then one morning, as I was seeing patients in the clinic, the discomfort in my chest intensified, and my left arm became very cold. Again, I cannot describe the feeling as one of pain, heaviness, or pressure; rather, it was a deep sense that something was just not right. It was at that moment I began to feel a profound "sense of impending doom."

I asked the clinic nurses to run an electrocardiogram on me. When I looked at it there were unmistakable signs of acute myocardial ischemia. The director of the catheterization laboratory happened to also be in clinic that morning and when I showed him the tracing he exclaimed, "You're having a heart attack! You're going to the cath lab right now!" I was then caught up in a whirlwind of activity, being rushed to the lab, intravenous lines started, medications given.

Somehow, I felt detached from the whole process, a sense that I was a distant observer of some great drama in progress. The catheterization revealed an 80 percent blockage of one major coronary and a 70 percent blockage in another, with a small branch vessel being totally occluded. Angioplasty and stent placement of the two major arteries soon followed, but the branch vessel could not be opened. A small part of my heart had died.

Later, as I lay in a hospital bed on the cardiology floor, I thought about what had just transpired. Clearly, the medical technology that I had always trusted had let me down. Had I believed the test results rather than my own instincts, then I very well may not have survived. I also realized how inadequate words are to describe angina and how easily it might go unnoticed by lay people. Technology is fine, but it has its limits, and has to be combined with clinical experience to be truly effective. What would have happened to a non-physician in the same situation? I doubt the outcome would have been as good.

I gazed out the window of my room into the night sky. The stars were coming out, and I could just barely see the thin crescent of the moon appear. The new moon! The Tarot reader had been right. Granted, she was six months off time-wise, but then again, the stress test wasn't that accurate, either. I smiled remembering her words, and realized that the universe is more mysterious and odd than I ever imagined.

It is said that there is a blessing for everything, and so there is a traditional blessing to be said on the coming of the new moon. Quietly, I recited the words of the ancient prayer, a heartfelt expression of gratitude: "Grant us a long life, a peaceful life of goodness and blessing, sustenance and health and let us say, Amen."

DANCING WITH THE CRAB

"Fear is the pain before the wound."
—*Noah ben Shea*

IT STARTED AS a spot on my neck. A slightly discolored area, I really did not pay much attention to it. Slowly however, it grew larger, taking on a progressively darker appearance. My wife grew concerned about it and began to pester me to get it looked at. One morning, as I arrived at the hospital, I met one of the dermatologists in the hallway. I nonchalantly asked, "Is this anything to worry about?" as I pulled my collar down to show her the area. She took one look at it and said, "Yes," then took my hand and said, "Come with me."

"Where are we going?" I asked. "For a biopsy," she replied. Despite my protests about things I had scheduled she would hear nothing of it. Within a few minutes, I was lying in the procedure room of the dermatology clinic getting lidocaine injected into my neck. Quickly and skillfully she snipped away a small piece of the area and sent it off to pathology.

"What do you think it is?" I asked. She hesitated for a long moment.

"Let's wait till the biopsy's back." By then my beeper was already going off, and I had to rush off to my morning clinic. The look on the dermatologist's face haunted me, but I tried to put it out of my mind. By the next day I could think of nothing else. I paged her several times but couldn't get through. Finally, after giving a lecture at another hospital I received a page from her. I answered from my car phone.

"The biopsy is back," she said. "I've had it checked twice." She hesitated for a moment. "It is a rare form of cancer, a type that can spread rapidly. You will need surgery, perhaps chemo and radiation." Another pause then, "I'm sorry ..."

The next five days were a blur. Reality sinks in only slowly and with it a growing sense of panic. The surgeon assures me he will keep dissecting till he has clean margins, while trying for a "cosmetically acceptable outcome." I have seen the results of neck surgeries before. I gaze into the mirror and imagine what I will look like, then turn away.

Cancer, the crab, so named because it spreads out like the multiple legs of a crab. Your own body gone wild, turning against you, a betrayal by yourself. You alternate between anger and fear, hope and despair. And yet, in the midst of it all, the world has somehow never seemed so full of wonder.

I soon found it increasingly difficult to sleep. Without sleep, everything, ambition, desire, hope, and fear, all slowly fade into an amorphous and murky haze. As my insomnia persisted, the lack of dreaming began to produce a weird sort of sensory distortion, with memories and pictures suddenly forming in my mind during the course of the day, often triggered by some random taste or smell. By the time the day of surgery finally arrived, I had reached an odd state somewhere beyond exhaustion, where everyday objects began to appear surreal and virtually pulse with color. Even the gray cloudy winter sky seemed to give off an intense and luminous glow.

When the surgery finally began, the feel of the sedatives gently overcoming my consciousness was almost a welcome relief. You hand your life over to the physicians and nurses around you, in a profound moment of both trust and resignation. Then, the darkness. When you return what you notice first is the pain. Calling like a beacon to summon you back from oblivion, the pain rises from a dull ache to a throbbing intensity. The whole world is pain. You finally come back enough to feel the source and try to reach for it, but something stops you. It is my wife's hand. Slowly, the world comes back into focus. Forms, shapes and colors reappear. My wife strokes my head and tells me that the surgeon had to cut wide and deep, but got all of it. They feel I am cured. I close my eyes and utter a silent prayer of thanks.

All things considered, the scar is not bad. But I cannot hide from it. There are certain wounds that will never fully heal, that somehow become incorporated into the very fabric of our souls. Each time I look into the mirror, its presence reminds me that there is always the chance it may some day recur, at some other time, in some other place (and that next time I might not be so lucky).

I spoke over dinner with a friend of mine, a breast cancer survivor, about this constant fear of a recurrence. She nodded knowingly. "Yes," she sighed. "At first you live each day on a tightrope, trying to balance hope and fear. Then, you slowly come to accept it, and eventually your cancer becomes a kind of partner in a strange sort of dance, always waiting for it to try and bite you again."

"A dance with the crab?" I asked.

"Yes," she smiled. "That's it; the rest of your life is spent dancing with the crab." And at that we laughed, raised our glasses and toasted, "L'chayim. To Life!"

SONGS FROM A DISTANT TIME

"Where words fail, music speaks."
—*Hans Christian Andersen*

J DREADED HAVING TO do this case. An 85-year-old woman had been transferred from her nursing home for a replacement of her failing pacemaker. The attendant who had helped transfer her to the hospital warned us that she suffered from advanced Alzheimer's disease, was frequently combative, and would become very agitated when given sedatives. When the nurses came near her, she would withdraw and repeatedly shout, "No, No!" over and over again. Several people tried to calmly explain to her what we were doing and why, but she would push them away and shout: "No!"

The gurney upon which she has been transported had been moved into the operating area but she refused to move off of it to the procedure table. Her agitation grew and she tried to strike the nurses around her. "No," she shouted again and again. "No!" The thought of trying to operate on a combative, demented woman, who did not yet have an intravenous line placed, did not enthrall me. Indeed, I was just about to cancel the case when a glimmer from the other side of the room caught my eye.

We had recently had a new sound system installed in the pacemaker suite, and a pile of CDs sat next to the audio player. I have always played music during procedures, finding it helps me, the staff and the patients relax. Almost without thinking, I walked over to the pile of CDs and picked up one entitled *The Best of the Big Band Era*, placed it in the machine and hit the play button. The room abruptly filled with the sounds of swing music, rich, full and pulsating with energy. Then, within moments of starting the music the most re-markable thing happened.

The old woman stopped screaming. She seemed transfixed, her eyes glazed over, seemingly focused on a place far away. She suddenly transformed into a quiet, cooperative, almost docile person. The nurses eased her over onto the operating table, placed an IV line and prepped her for the procedure. All the while she did not move or speak. It was as if the music flowing through the room had cast a spell on her. Heeding the warning from the nursing home, I decided not to give her any sedative and perform the procedure under local anesthesia only. As I made the first incision, the woman did not move or utter a word, still transfixed by the pulsating music.

Then after a few minutes had passed an even more remarkable thing occurred. She began to speak. In a surprisingly clear resonant voice, words seemed to tumble out of her. "He was so handsome," she said, "I didn't think he had even noticed me. I was shocked when he asked me to dance. I felt like I was flying."

She spoke on and on, about the music, the war, her love for dancing, and her long-dead husband. At one point during the procedure, I thought she was trying to move, then I realized she was tapping her foot in time to the infectious rhythms of the melody that pulsated through the room.

The response of the nurses to her transformation was equally remarkable. They went from screaming at her when she first arrived to gently stroking her head and whispering softly, "It is almost over, Mary, you're doing great." Shortly thereafter, I finished the procedure and the nurses removed the drapes and moved her to the postoperative area, making sure that the music went with her. As opposed to when she arrived, she lay on the gurney peaceful and smiling, her head nodding in time to the sounds of Benny Goodman and Jimmy Dorsey. Afterwards I stood there, looking at the woman and contemplating what had just occurred.

The music had managed to reach deep into the mind of this woman, beyond the neurofilrillary amyloid tangles of Alzheimer's that had clogged her brain to the part that held precious memories of her youth. Researchers have shown that music seems to function as a kind of a language, one that speaks directly to the emotional areas of the brain. According to the noted musicologist David Tame, "Music is more than a language, it is the language of languages. It can be said that of all the arts, there is none other that more powerfully moves and changes the consciousness." Recent studies have suggested that music communicates information capable of provoking a specific emotional response in the brain and is able to do so despite the differences in a person's personality, culture, taste or training. As such, music may be as uniquely human a form of communication as is spoken language, perhaps even more so.

When the attendants from the nursing home arrived to take the woman back, they were amazed at how tranquil she was. When I told them what had occurred, they could not believe it, stating that she had hardly spoken in years. As they were starting to leave I stood by the gurney and gently touched the woman's hand. She turned her head, her eyes looking deep into mine and smiled.

VOICES

"There are more things in heaven and earth, Horatio, than are dreamt of in your philosophy."
—Shakespeare, Hamlet, Act 1, Scene 5

I HAVE ALWAYS BEEN puzzled by it. My father was not a man given to speculation of things outside the confines of day-to-day life. The horrors of spending years in front-line combat in World War II destroyed any belief he might have had in religion or the paranormal. He lived his life in a hard state of bitter melancholy, his workaholic lifestyle a balm to blot out the pain of the past. That is what made the incident even more perplexing. My father adored my uncle Bill, seeing in him the figure of the father he himself had never known. Bill was elderly, living alone in a small yet tidy apartment. One night, after arising from sleep to visit the bathroom, he fell, striking the floor with such force that he was unable to move from the bathroom. A searing pain ran through his left hip, causing him to cry out in agony.

Miles away, my father suddenly awoke from a sound sleep. Waking my mother, he said, "Something is wrong with Bill." My mother tried to assure him that it had just been a bad dream. My father would hear nothing of it and proceeded to call Bill's apartment by phone. When he failed to answer, both my parents became alarmed. They got dressed and drove to Bill's apartment and upon entering found him lying nearly unconscious on the bathroom floor. He had broken a hip and had hemorrhaged a large amount of blood into the area. He was taken by ambulance to a nearby hospital. The physicians who cared for Bill said that if he had lain there much longer he would not have survived. Whenever I asked my father about it he would look somewhat embarrassed and shrug his shoulders, quietly saying, "A voice."

My mother-in-law was a hard, often-bitter woman who resented the lack of opportunity and the confinement that her life had provided. She was staunchly anti-religion and believed only in what she could see, smell and taste. Yet when my wife suddenly became seriously ill while at college, and was whisked away to a hospital before anyone could call, an odd thing occurred. My mother-in-law abruptly awoke from a sound sleep. Waking her husband, she exclaimed, "Something is wrong with Barbara!" Her husband tried to assure her it was just a bad dream, but she persisted. Just then, the phone rang; the hospital was calling to inform them that my wife had arrived in the emergency room. When asked about it afterward, she would shrug her shoulders and shake her head, saying, "I heard a voice."

In the 1960s and 1970s, the concept of telepathy (Extra Sensory Perception or ESP, as it was re-named) became the focus of intense scientific inquiry, principally conducted by the U.S. military. For the most part, while the claims of ESP were largely dismissed, investigators found a number of substantiated instances that just could not be explained, cases like those of my father and mother-in-law, where voices came in the dead of night.

I think of this now as I finish speaking to the family of a man recently recovered from a cardiac arrest. The man had collapsed at home and was found by his son, only after the son suddenly awoke from a sound sleep sensing something was terribly wrong with his father. When I asked the son how he knew, he merely shrugged his shoulders and shook his head, saying, "I don't know, it was like a voice or something."

I have always struggled with such things. The scientist in me wants to dismiss them as coincidence while another part of me cannot yet help but wonder. Maybe we are all in some way connected, in a manner we cannot yet begin to understand. And perhaps, just perhaps, we can, on rare occasions, hear the voice of a beloved soul in distress, calling out to another.

REKINDLING THE FLAME

I REALLY DIDN'T THINK she was going to make it. Once a bouncy and perky 7-year-old girl who loved more than anything to dance, she slowly began to lose her stamina. With each passing day she seemed to grow more and more weak and fatigued. When she suddenly awoke in the night saying she could no longer breathe, she was rushed to the local hospital. There she was found to be in florid congestive heart failure with a barely beating heart that virtually filled the whole of her chest. She was transported by helicopter to us in the middle of the night as a potential transplant candidate. She was near death when she came. However, on arrival we found her to be in a sustained idiopathic ventricular tachycardia that appeared to be coming from the left ventricle, which had dilated her heart to a barely contracting mass of tissue. We stabilized her heart failure, but we could not keep her out of the tachycardia despite our best attempts at drug therapy.

This was over a decade ago and radiofrequency ablation had just been introduced and was still considered highly experimental. We offered this to the parents as a way to stop this incessant rhythm that was destroying her heart, and with teary eyes they agreed to let us try. When I spoke to Emily, the little girl, her only question was "Will I be able to dance?"

The next day we took her to the lab and slowly and methodically mapped the tachycardia. Finally, after what seemed to be forever, we found a suitable target site. Holding the catheter tightly, with my own heart pounding in my chest, I ordered the energy turned on. The tachycardia that had nearly taken her life and had proven so resistant to therapy disappeared in an instant. For the first time in weeks her heart maintained its normal rhythm. For the briefest of moments, I felt a surge of sheer joy, but then quickly repressed it. "It may come back," I thought. "She may have complications, the failure may not resolve." When I spoke to her parents I dampened my words with phrases like "might be gone," and "we'll have to see what happens," always hedging my bets against possible failure. Again for the briefest of moments I saw a flicker of fire within them, but my cautious words quickly extinguished it. The flame of passion was once again put out by my own fear of being burnt by it.

Later that day when the child was awake and back in her room I returned to check on her. Her little eyes were bright and her smile reached from ear to ear. "Am I fixed?" she asked, the words virtually bubbling out of her. The room was filled with family, and I again put on my reserved and cool exterior, remembering all too well the times in the past when things had not gone as expected, and muttered a somewhat restrained, "Yes, I hope so." Her bright little eyes then seemed to stare into my very soul, and her innocent voice asked, "Then why aren't you happy?"

I froze, not knowing what to say, for she had touched on the very question that all of us struggling with the strain of the ever shifting landscape of modern medicine must come to face: What became of our passion, the flame that once seemed to burn so brightly within us? Only by recognizing those emotional instances that lie hidden in the daily moments of our work do we come to understand the conflict that rages within each of us, our longing for the creative and passionate internal fire with its wondrous warmth and intensity, balanced with our innate fear of being burnt by it. The brilliant poet and philosopher David Whyte says that finding this fire is an essential need for preserving a person's soul, for, "while we believe we are merely going to work each day to earn a living, the soul is secretly locked in a life-or-death struggle for its own survival." Yet at the very moment, when the fire begins to glow within us, the fear comes over us. Our memories fill with every complication, bad outcome, or lawsuit that we have seen or experienced.

Whyte describes these critical moments as when "the universe turns toward us, realizing we are here and about to make our mark. We hear the wild divine elements in the world hold their breath, waiting for our next move, our next word, but at last the center of real attention, we turn and take a step back ..." Whyte goes on to say, "that being afraid of the fire and the possibility of being burnt, we freeze everything and everyone around us so they can neither move nor feel the warmth of their own flames, that we reject those wondrous moments that offer the soul a chance for complete fulfillment. It is difficult to experience joy, the risks seem just too great and its occurrence at work may be so powerful that we can experience it as a sense of terror." We somehow prefer to be in a "comfortably numb" state of self-anesthesia with which we are more familiar.

Yet there is no choice without consequences, for we simply cannot ignore our soul's fire without damaging ourselves in the process. A vital passion still smolders within us, regardless of whether it is acknowledged or not. Failing to allow the fire to come forth, our souls fill with a dense toxic smoke, like a flame starved for oxygen. This poisonous smog is composed of complaint, blame, resentment and self-pity. The longer we ignore it, the more we are overcome with its noxious components. Whyte states that we need only open ourselves for a moment to the fresh air of the world for this smoldering mass to burst into a flame with the power to transform the ordinary into the exquisite and wondrous.

All this passed through my mind in an eternal instant. I felt myself relax, as if this child had somehow cast an immense burden from me. Our attention was then drawn to the flickering television screen perched just above our heads. The children's channel was playing *Cinderella*, and the story was just at the point where Prince Charming asks the beautiful young lady who has caught his eye to dance.

Emily turned to me and asked, "Will I be able to dance?" In answer I bent down and swept the child up into my arms. Then with her suspended in air, we slowly waltzed around the room to the music, as her family clapped and Emily giggled with delight.

THE NAME

I HAVE ALWAYS BEEN fascinated by names. While a "rose by any other name would smell as sweet," a name nonetheless seems to play a surprisingly important role in how we define a place, person or a moment. Language is one of mankind's greatest of inventions and one of the first tasks of language is to assign names to things in the vast world around us, making order out of the apparent chaos. Indeed, in many cultures, names of people are felt to possess a significant power over their lives and are chosen with great care, often to honor some person or event.

All of this was far from my mind as I arrived to start what I thought was to be a routine placement of a pacemaker in an elderly patient. A new representative from the pacemaker company was present and after a brief introduction I realized that we had met before, many years ago.

She had been young and enthusiastic and eager to work. She was hired by a prominent, highly skilled surgeon who treated her kindly and taught her how to work in a medical office. A gentle, dignified, scholarly and religious man, she looked upon him as an inspiring mentor. Years passed and she had been in her last months of pregnancy when she received word that the surgeon had suffered a massive heart attack and was being rushed to the medical school hospital. He was in cardiogenic shock when he arrived. By chance I was the cardiologist on call that evening. After being rushed to the catheterization laboratory, the interventional cardiologist managed to get the occluded vessels open again, a difficult task in that pre-stent era. He initially stabilized only to once again go into shock, forcing a late-night return to the catheterization laboratory for a repeat intervention. I remained with him throughout the night; his condition was too unstable to be left to the house staff to manage. By late morning his condition had finally stabilized. The young pregnant woman had been there through much of the ordeal, and when it was finally over, between sighs of relief and utterances of thanks, she said, "I won't forget you." Physicians in the aftermath of crisis often hear such things, but seldom does anything seem to come of it. Our encounters with patients and their loved ones are all too frequently tangential, fleeting and quickly forgotten. The hectic nature of medicine soon resumed and the event faded from my mind.

Now, years later, the woman's presence in the pacemaker suite had triggered a flood of memories of that night long ago. She was insistent on showing me a recent picture of the child she had carried at the time. She produced a color photograph of a handsome bright-eyed boy with a wide grin.

"What's his name?" I asked.

"His name?" she replied and after a brief pause said, "His name is Blair ..."

For a long moment I stood in utter silence, unsure of what to say or do, then slowly leaned forward to kiss her forehead and utter "Thank you."

THE HARVEST

*I*T STARTED WITH pain in my arms, followed by weakness. As it progressed, I became increasingly concerned and had a magnetic resonance imaging of cervical spine performed. The technician who performed the scan had a grave look on her face and did not want me to leave until a neurologist had looked at the films. Puzzled, I called one of the neurologists I knew and asked him to come over. Upon looking at the films, a look of concern came over his face as well.

"The C6-C7 disc is completely displaced and compressing your spinal cord." While he thought I would probably need surgery, he suggested that I begin physical therapy to see whether the disc might slide back into place.

In physical therapy, I was placed in traction. A collar is positioned around my neck and jaw and attached to a counter-weight designed to stretch my neck and expand the space between the vertebrae, encouraging the disc to slip back into place. While reasonably safe and effective, there is a small chance that an unstable disc may rupture under traction, allowing its contents to push outward and acutely compress the cord. After the traction device is removed, I go to begin my clinic when suddenly I start to feel quite odd. Within a short period of time, my pen starts to fall out of my hands. I begin dropping cups and then have trouble holding charts. My arms and legs turn numb and wobble when I try to walk. I nervously page the physician director of physical therapy who immediately comes to see me. After a careful examination, he looks at me and says "You are developing an acute cord compression syndrome, you need surgery, now."

Suddenly I go from doctor to patient, from vertical to horizontal, while the physical therapy director begins making frantic phone calls to my internist and neurologist. I become caught in a whirlwind of activity. The neurosurgeon who was contacted wants me moved from the University Hospital to a large nearby private hospital where special equipment is available. After I arrive, there is a flurry of activity, blood draws, x-rays, IV's started and high-dose steroids given. The neurosurgeon comes by to see me. He seems quite young, but speaks in a confident and straightforward manner. I feel like I know him from somewhere, but cannot quite place him. As opposed to most surgeons, his manner is relaxed yet focused. He answers all of the questions that my wife and I ask in a thorough, straightforward, yet caring manner. I still feel like I knew him from somewhere. I have the same déja vu-like sensation when I meet the anesthesiologist and the physician's assistant, both of whom seem efficient and caring.

A confrontation with serious illness often provokes a period of deep self-reflection and examination. I had spent my career in academia, much of it teaching residents, fellows, medical students, nurses and physician assistants. The very real fear that I might end up paralyzed and disabled made me wonder, did I make the right choice? Would my family have been better off if I had gone into the more lucrative world of private practice? Did the students and the residents learn anything from me? Did all those years of effort really matter?

My condition steadily worsens. I begin to lose motor control and start having spontaneous contractions of muscles all over my body (a condition referred to as "spinal myoclonus"). As I am being taken to the operating room I continue to have the feeling that I know many of the staff around me, even though I am in a hospital different from my own.

Entering the operating room, the anesthesiologist has a concerned look on his face. Due to the instability of my neck he chooses to intubate me in a semi-awake state (fiber-optic intubation). Although the surgery is originally projected to take an hour, it lasts more than four hours.

When I awake in the recovery area, my wife is holding my hand and my neck is very sore. The anesthesiologist comes by to check on me and remarks "You may not remember me, but I was a resident under you many years ago." I offer a groggy word of thanks and shake his hand. Then, after I return to my room, one after the other a procession of nurses, physician assistants and physicians (even my surgeon) come by to tell me that I had once taught them in medical, nursing or physicians assistant school, or as residents and fellows. I was surrounded by people that I had once helped train! I had once taught them how to take care of patients and now they were taking care of me. Things had come full circle, in a cycle as old as time itself. It is written, "As you sow so shall you reap."

All physicians will one day be patients. I now know that for those who have devoted themselves over the years to the education and training of students, interns, residents and fellows that there will come a time when we shall harvest the seeds of knowledge and caring that we have so carefully sown. And when we do it will be a good harvest. A harvest of plenty.

A PSALM FOR SOULS DEPARTED

ON AUGUST 19, 1998, MY FATHER died. The sudden and unexpected nature of the event threw my already-hectic life into a state of disruption that only now has dissipated. Now, exactly one year later, in accordance with custom, the family gathered together again to place the headstone that would mark his grave. As opposed to the funeral, during which the weather was unbearably hot and humid, the day was cool and pleasant and the sky a clear deep blue.

I, however, was in a somber mood as we approached the site. The year since his death had been difficult for all of us. The heavy demands of being a physician had often impeded my attempts at recitation of the mourner's prayer (the Kaddish) that a son should say over the course of a year in memory of a father (the needs of the living outweighing the needs of the dead). Sorting out the numerous tax and financial problems left by his passing had also been difficult and frustrating.

Suddenly, the usual silence of the cemetery was shattered by the least expected of sounds, the deep and resonant tones of a pipe organ. An organ? Here? I whirled around to face the direction of the sound and was astounded to find a single man, seated in a small amphitheater (usually used for funerals), playing the largest accordion I have ever seen. One often thinks of the accordion as an instrument of light, airy, polka-like pieces. Yet the notes were deep, full and resonant, echoing off the acoustic backdrop of the amphitheater, making the instrument sound like a massive pipe organ. I recognized the piece, Bach's "Little" fugue in G minor. I was entranced, immobile, and unable to speak as the sheer force of the music passed over me. This was not a frivolous act. The very soul of the player seemed to flow through the complex melody with a reverence and emotion that I have seldom heard. I was puzzled at first until a realization came over me that while others had brought flowers (as Asians bring rice) to honor the memory of the departed, he had brought music and with it a sense of sanctification to this place.

The scattered people there that morning, as if drawn by some unspoken command, slowly gathered around the amphitheater. The man, who appeared to be in his late 40s, was oblivious to our presence. I had never dreamt an accordion could make such music. He played another Bach piece and then launched into sections of Mozart's magnificent "Requiem." A guard approached, appearing intent on stopping him. Almost in unison, the crowd of people turned and glared at him. The guard stopped, hesitated for a moment, turned and walked away. The mysterious player then launched into his last piece, which I did not recognize. It was a melodious, soaringly beautiful piece, played with a blend of emotion and reverence that I had never heard before (or since). As he played, tears rolled down his face and down our faces as well. At the piece's soaring finale he seemed to collapse in a sweat-drenched state of exhaustion. The crowd applauded but he appeared not to hear. He wept.

As the others dispersed, I went up and sat next to him on one of the amphitheater's benches. "It was wonderful," I said. He nodded his head in silent acknowledgement. After a long moment, he told me he was a professional musician, a concert pianist, composer and arranger. His father, a refugee from war-ravaged Europe, had a particular fondness for the accordion (especially when used in polka and klezmer music), and played the instrument reasonably well. His father had begged him to play the accordion, but he rejected it, feeling it incapable of "real" music.

Years went by and he became an accomplished and respected musician. His father would always tease him, "So why can't you learn to play something on the accordion?" He ignored him. Then, like my father, his father died suddenly without a chance to say goodbye. In his will he bequeathed him his accordion. At first he could not bear to look at it, but one day he picked it up and decided to try to play it.

Over the next several years he had thrown himself into mastering the instrument with a near-manic intensity, exploring its subtleties and nuances. He decided to push its limits, to try to elicit sounds from it that no one else had yet found. Finally, he had composed the last piece he had played, "A Psalm for Souls Departed." Today he had played it for his father, whose grave was located just across from the amphitheater, and for all the departed souls whose memories dwell in this place. "I hope he heard," the man said. "I am sure he heard," I replied, "and I am sure he is quite proud."

I rose, shook his hand, and returned to my father's graveside. But, now my mood was no longer somber, for the music had somehow uplifted and transformed it into something different. Indeed, something wondrous and transcendent seemed to fill the entire place, giving it a wondrous almost radiant beauty.

"Magnified and sanctified," I said, losing myself in the words of the ancient mourner's prayer, "may his great name be blessed."

"Above all blessings and hymns and praises and consolations that are uttered in the world," I intoned, remembering the beauty of the music that had been the musician's prayer, "may his great name be blessed.

"May a great peace from heaven, and life, be upon us all, and let us all say Amen."

GLOSSARY OF MEDICAL TERMS

Arrhythmia: loss or abnormality of rhythm, especially an irregularity of the heart beat.

Atrial fibrillation (Atrial flutter): an irregular and at times very rapid abnormal heart rhythm.

Atrioventricular nodal ablation: A procedure in which a special catheter is guided up into the heart via an insertion point in the groin. The head of the catheter has electrical sensors, which help the cardiologist to guide the catheter to the correct place. Once the catheter is in place the cardiologist can deliver electrical pulses, which destroy (ablate) the tissue that is causing the heart problem.

Basal rates: a steady trickle of low levels of longer-acting insulin, such as that used in insulin pumps.

Beta-blocker: a medicine used to treat various cardiovascular diseases that acts by blocking receptors at nerve endings.

Cardiogenic shock: a state in which a weakened heart is not able to pump enough blood to meet the body's needs, often resulting in death.

Cardiomyopathy: literally means "heart muscle disease"; is the deterioration of the function of the myocardium (i.e., the actual heart muscle) such that it does not pump blood normally.

Catheterization: passage of a catheter, a tubular instrument to allow passage of fluid from or into a body cavity or blood vessel.

Congestive heart failure: the inability of the heart to adequately pump enough blood to meet the body's needs.

Coronary: refers to the arteries that supply the heart with blood.

CPR: cardiopulmonary resuscitation

Diffuse ST segments: changes in an electrocardiogram that indicate a heart attack could be occurring.

ECG (also, EKG): electrocardiogram, a recording of the electrical activity of the heart.

EP Study: a test done to evaluate the heart's electrical conduction system by inserting small catheters into the heart and reproducing symptoms and rhythm disturbances in a controlled setting.

Esophageal spasm: irregular or abnormal contractions of the muscles in the esophagus.

Endotracheal tube: a tube placed with the trachea, a tube-like portion of the breathing or "respiratory" tract that connects the "voice box" (larynx) with the bronchial parts of the lungs.

Extubate: to remove a tube from an organ, structure or orifice; specifically, removal of the endotracheal tube after intubation.

Glioma: A brain tumor that begins in a glial, or supportive, cell, in the brain or spinal cord. One of the most malignant tumors that exist, they are usually fatal.

Holters: a continuous EKG recording system that a patient wears overnight.

Hypertrophic cardiomyopathy: A disease of the myocardium (the muscle of the heart) in which a portion of the myocardium is hypertrophied (thickened) without any obvious cause. A common cause of sudden death in young people.

Implantable defibrillator: A very small electronic device, the automatic defibrillator is inserted below the collarbone of patients and can correct life-threatening irregular heartbeat problems, called arrhythmias. An electric shock delivered through tiny electrodes on the heart help correct the rhythm and prevent death.

Leiomyosarcoma: a tumor of smooth muscle often in the small intestine.

Long QT syndrome: a disorder of the heart's electrical activity that may cause one to develop a sudden, uncontrollable and dangerous heart rhythm disorder resulting in death. In one form (LQT2) strong emotions may provoke potentially lethal events.

Myocardial ischemia: decreased blood flow to the heart caused by constriction or obstruction of an artery.

Neurofilrillary amyloid tangle: Amyloid is a general term for protein fragments that the body produces normally. Neurofibrillary tangles are insoluble twisted fibers found inside the brain's cells. These tangles consist primarily of a protein called tau. In Alzheimer's disease, however, the tau protein is abnormal and the microtubule structures collapse, accumulating in the brain.

Peripheral edema: Edema is observable swelling from fluid accumulation in body tissues. Edema most commonly occurs in the feet and legs, where it is referred to as peripheral edema. Often a sign of heart failure.

QRS complexes: the deflections in the tracing of the electrocardiogram (ECG or EKG), comprising the Q, R, and S waves that represent the ventricular activity of the heart (the depolarization of the ventricles).

Radiofrequency ablation: a minimally invasive, targeted treatment in which a catheter — attached to a device that delivers radiofrequency (RF) energy — is inserted into the heart. The RF energy is then applied to heat and destroy abnormal tissue that causes disturbances in the hearts normal rhythm thereby curing the disorder.

S3gallop: an accentuated third heart sound in patients with cardiac disease.

Senning repair: a surgical procedure used to repair the congenital heart malformation referred to as D-transposition of the great vessels.

Sick sinus syndrome: abnormal functioning of the structure that regulates the heartbeat, causing episodes of abnormal heart rhythm.

Spina bifida: a birth defect in which there is a bony defect in the vertebral column so that part of the spinal cord, which is normally protected within the vertebral column, is exposed.

Sustained idiopathic ventricular tachycardia: a fast, potentially life-threatening heart rhythm lasting for more than thirty seconds.

Transposition: the condition of being in the wrong place or on the wrong side of the body.

Transposition of the great vessels: a malformation in which the aorta and pulmonary artery are in two separate and parallel circulations.

Ventricular fibrillation: a condition in which disordered electrical activity causes the ventricles of the heart to contract in a rapid, unsynchronized, uncoordinated fashion, resulting in death.